the Macrobiotic Cancer Prevention Cookbook

the Macrobiotic Cancer Prevention Cookbook

Aveline Kushi
with
Wendy Esko

AVERY PUBLISHING GROUP INC.
Garden City Park, New York

The medical and health procedures in this book are based on the training, personal experiences, and research of the author. Because each person and situation is unique, the editor and publisher urge the reader to check with a qualified health professional before using any procedure where there is any question as to its appropriateness.

The publisher does not advocate the use of any particular diet and exercise program, but believes the information presented in this book should be available to the public.

Because there is always some risk involved, the author and publisher are not responsible for any adverse effects or consequences resulting from the use of any of the suggestions, preparations, or procedures in this book. Please do not use the book if you are unwilling to assume the risk. Feel free to consult a physician or other qualified health professional. It is a sign of wisdom, not cowardice, to seek a second or third opinion.

Cover Design: Rudy Shur and Martin Hochberg
In-House Editors: Nancy Marks Papritz and Diana Puglisi
Typesetter: Multifacit Graphics, Inc.

Library of Congress Cataloging in Publication Data

Kushi, Aveline.
     The macrobiotic cancer prevention cookbook / Aveline Kushi
with Wendy Esko.
     p.   cm.
    Bibliography: p.
    Includes index.
    ISBN 0-89529-391-9
     1. Cancer—Prevention. 2. Cancer—Diet Therapy—Recipes.
   3. Macrobiotic diet—Recipes. I. Esko, Wendy. II. Title.
   RC268.K87 1988
641.5′631—dc19
                                          88-24250
                                                 CIP

Printed in the United States of America

10 9 8 7 6 5

Contents

Acknowledgements

We would like to thank everyone who inspired and contributed to this cookbook.

We would like to thank Michio Kushi for his untiring dedication to creating a healthy and peaceful world, and for pioneering the macrobiotic dietary and lifestyle approach to preventing cancer, heart disease, and other degenerative disorders of the twentieth century.

We also thank Edward Esko for guidance and inspiration in organizing and completing the book, and extend appreciation to Alex Jack for reviewing the text and offering suggestions and advice.

We also thank Rudy Shur, Steve Blauer, Diana Puglisi, Nancy Marks Papritz, and our other friends at Avery Publishing Group for their help in transforming the idea for this book into reality.

We also extend our deepest gratitude to George and Lima Ohsawa, who introduced modern macrobiotics throughout the world, and to our millions of macrobiotic friends in East and West, and North and South who are daily living a healthier and more peaceful way of life.

Aveline Kushi
Wendy Esko

Preface

As a child in pre-war Japan, the problem of cancer was very remote. I can't remember anyone in my small mountain village or in my family developing it. Of course, our rural diet was traditionally-based and more natural than today. It was not until I came to this country years later that I encountered steak, ice cream, soft drinks—and the modern epidemic of cancer.

When my husband Michio and I began teaching more than thirty years ago, our main concern was to introduce everyone to a more healthful, natural diet, and to secure the highest quality foods. We began asking farmers to grow organic brown rice and other whole grains, and made arrangements with traditional food processors in Japan to ship high-quality miso, tamari soy sauce, sea-vegetables, and other natural foods to the United States. We also encouraged our students and friends to use fresh organic vegetables and fruits. At that time, I had no idea that researchers would eventually discover that many of these foods had specific properties that reduced the risk of cancer.

As the natural food movement grew from these small beginnings, I began to realize that cancer had become a major problem that threatened modern civilization. I also began to understand that an extreme or unbalanced diet contributed to cancer, and that macrobiotic lifestyle and dietary practice offered everyone the hope of preventing it. At this time, Michio and I started to discuss the relationship between diet and cancer in our lectures and seminars, and encouraged our macrobiotic educational organizations to focus on this theme as well. Soon afterward, the East West Foundation arranged the first in a series of yearly conferences on cancer and diet, and published several reports on this subject. These conferences were attended by many doctors and researchers, and by people who had recovered their health through macrobiotic lifestyle and dietary practice.

In the twelve years since these efforts began, there has been a tremendous growth in awareness of the relationship between diet, lifestyle, and cancer. Practically every week we read new reports linking some aspect of the modern diet and way of life with cancer. Leading public health organizations have begun to issue warnings about the modern diet, and have made dietary recommendations for preventing cancer that are remarkably similiar to those we have been recommending in macrobiotic dietary practice.

Many of the foods used daily in macrobiotic cooking have been shown to protect people from cancer. Whole grains, the staple in macrobiotic kitchens, contain beneficial fiber, which reduces the risk of cancer of the colon. In a study conducted in Japan, miso, a traditional seasoning for soups and other dishes, was shown to lower the risk of stomach cancer, while other studies have shown that sea-vegetables, also a part of the macrobiotic diet, inhibit the development of tumors. Moreover, orange-yellow vegetables, such as squash, carrots, and others containing beta-carotene, have also been shown to lower the risk of cancer.

In this introductory book, we explain how to use these and other whole natural foods as a part of a balanced diet and way of life. We offer guidelines for selecting the highest quality natural foods, advice on setting up your kitchen, and helpful hints on menu planning and getting started. In the recipe section, we offer complete natural food menus for one week. As you will discover in these pages, healthful eating can be delicious and fun.

I would like to thank Wendy Esko, who with the help of her husband, Edward, gathered the material for this book and arranged it in its present form. I also thank my husband, Michio, for contributing the Foreword, and for his untiring dedication to the dream of world health and world peace. I also thank Alex Jack, co-author with Michio of the *Cancer Prevention Diet* (St. Martin's Press, 1983), for reviewing the text and making helpful suggestions. I appreciate the guidance of our friends at Avery Publishing Group, including Rudy Shur, Stephen Blauer, Diana Puglisi, and Nancy Marks Papritz.

In closing, it is my hope that all of you who read this book will discover the joys of cooking with whole natural foods, and enjoy good health throughout life.

Aveline Kushi
Brookline, Massachusetts

Foreword

During the twentieth century, humanity has experienced the rise of modern degenerative diseases. As the modern diet and way of life have spread to all corners of the world, so have cancer, heart disease, diabetes, arthritis, and immune deficiencies. The increase in degenerative diseases has taken place even as medical science and technology have continued to develop.

When I came to this country nearly forty years ago, cancer affected about one person in seven. Now, it is estimated that one out of three will develop it, and in 1988, the American Cancer Society announced that one million new cases could be expected before the end of the year. Moreover, during the past ten years, the rate of melanoma, a virulent form of skin cancer, almost doubled, while breast cancer, which affected one woman in thirteen a decade ago, now affects one in ten.

As a result of these statistics, and of the personal suffering caused by cancer, people everywhere—both within the medical profession and outside of it—are seeking approaches to prevention. Among the possible avenues of prevention, a change in diet and lifestyle could offer the best hope of reversing these trends.

Evidence linking the modern diet with cancer continues to mount. In 1977, the United States Senate Select Committee on Nutrition and Human Needs reviewed the evidence and issued a landmark report entitled, *Dietary Goals for the United States*. The Committee suggested that dietary modification—especially increasing the consumption of complex carbohydrates, such as whole cereal grains, beans, and fresh local vegetables, and reducing the intake of saturated fat, cholesterol, and refined sugar—could lower the risk of cancer and other chronic diseases. These recommendations parallel those of macrobiotics.

These conclusions were echoed in 1982 in the National Academy of Sciences' report, *Diet, Nutrition and Cancer*. After reviewing the data linking diet and cancer, the Academy issued interim dietary guidelines that were similiar to those in *Dietary Goals*.

The key to cancer prevention lies in the kitchen. For more than thirty years, my wife Aveline and her associates have taught a traditional approach to food and cooking that fulfills the dietary guidelines of these and other public health agencies. This approach, known throughout the world as macrobiotics, is based on the use of whole cereal grains, beans and bean products, fresh local vegetables and fruits, sea-vegetables, and other whole natural foods. The macrobiotic way of eating, which is low in fat and high in complex carbohydrates and fiber, has successfully—and enjoyably—been adopted by hundreds of thousands of individuals and families.

Today, many people would agree that a naturally-balanced diet can lower their risk of cancer. However, without practical guidance on cooking and food selection, many people have difficulty changing their way of eating. This introductory book provides this much-needed guidance and fulfills the urgent need for practical instruction in applying preventive dietary guidelines at home in the kitchen.

I wish to thank Aveline for developing the menus, recipes, and approach to cooking macrobiotically presented in this and her other books. I also thank Wendy Esko, who is a well-known author, teacher of macrobiotic cooking, and mother of seven children, for working with Aveline in compiling the recipes and other materials contained in these pages.

The dream of a healthy and fulfilling life belongs to everyone. It is my hope that this introductory book will help guide everyone toward realizing this dream, and bring humanity one step closer to a world in which health and peace are enjoyed by all.

Michio Kushi
Brookline, Massachusetts

Chapter One
DIET AND CANCER

Nearly forty years have passed since my husband Michio and I came to America with the dream of creating health and peace throughout the world. From its modern beginnings, macrobiotics has always been inspired by the vision of planetary harmony. We began to teach in New York City, and later moved to Boston and established an educational center there. Today, there are macrobiotic centers in most of the major cities in North America and around the world.

In the beginning, one of our main concerns was making natural food available to the public. More than twenty years ago, we started Erewhon, a small natural food store in downtown Boston, to fulfill this need. From this modest beginning, Erewhon grew into one of the world's leading distributors of high-quality natural food, and helped launch the natural food movement. By Erewhon's tenth anniversary, nearly 10,000 natural food stores and cooperatives in North America were making whole grains, beans, organic produce, and items such as tofu, tamari soy sauce, miso, and sea-vegetables available to the public.

By the early 70s, the natural food movement had begun to change America's eating habits for the better. It was time to focus attention on the modern health crisis. We selected cancer as a symbol of the modern decline in health, and Michio began to lecture in Boston and around the world on the relationship between cancer and diet. He also presented the stories of people who had applied the principles of macrobiotics in their recovery from cancer. Meanwhile, the East West Foundation, a nonprofit educational organization that we started, arranged conferences and published reports that focused on this problem.

These activities started at a time when greater nutrition awareness was developing among people everywhere. In 1977, the Senate Select Committee on Nutrition and Human Needs published a report entitled *Dietary Goals for the United States*. The Select Committee had sponsored hearings at which leading doctors, nutritionists, and public health experts testified, and had come to the conclusion that the modern diet was a major factor in cancer, heart disease, and other chronic illnesses. The Select Committee made dietary recommendations for lowering the risk of these illnesses, and advised all Americans to reduce their consumption of saturated fat, sugar, and processed foods, and to increase their intake of complex carbohydrates such as whole grains, beans, and fresh vegetables. These dietary guidelines paralleled the macrobiotic way of eating.

A little more than five years later, the National Academy of Sciences published a landmark report, *Diet, Nutrition and Cancer*, which said that the modern diet was a major risk factor in the most common types of cancer. Like the Senate Select Committee, the academy issued dietary guidelines for lowering the risk of cancer. Again, these recommendations paralleled macrobiotics.

Some progress has been made, but more changes are necessary. In May 1986, the *New England Journal of Medicine* published an article entitled "Progress Against Cancer," which described how cancer is viewed among those in the medical field. The authors stated, "We are losing the war against cancer, notwithstanding progress against several uncommon forms of the disease, improvements in palliation, and extension of the productive years of life. A shift in research emphasis, from research on treatment to research on prevention, seems necessary if substantial progress against cancer is to be forthcoming."

What direction should cancer prevention research take? Increasingly, scientific evidence is pointing to the modern diet as a leading risk factor in the development of cancer, and toward a naturally balanced diet along the lines of macrobiotics as a key factor in preventing the disease. Macrobiotic educators have essentially been saying the same thing—that diet is important—for more than thirty years, both in the United States and around the world.

In this book, we show how the macrobiotic way of eating is consistent with the dietary guidelines for cancer prevention put forth by leading public health agencies. Moreover, we present a practical approach to applying these guidelines at home in the kitchen. As you will discover in these pages, eating healthfully can be fun and enjoyable. When prepared with style and imagination, whole natural foods are appetizing and delicious.

In the rest of this chapter, we will examine features of cancer prevention diets, both traditional and modern. We will also be creating a framework for your understanding of macrobiotics, because the features we discuss here are all things that traditional preventive diets have in common with the macrobiotic way of selecting and preparing foods.

PREVENTIVE DIETS COMPLEMENT OUR PHYSICAL STRUCTURE

The structure and arrangement of the teeth provide a clue to the ideal pattern of human nourishment. We have thirty-two adult teeth. Of these, twenty are molars or premolars. These grinding machines (the word "molar" is from the Latin word meaning "millstone") are ideal for crushing the tough plant fibers that are found in whole cereal grains, beans, seeds, and other complex carbohydrate foods.

There are also eight front incisor and four canine teeth. The word "incisor" comes from the Latin word meaning "to cut into," and these teeth are well suited for cutting vegetables. The four canine teeth can be used in tearing animal foods, but are not sharply pointed in everyone. People who live in societies that consume little animal food often do not develop pointed canines.

Using the teeth as a model, we can conclude that, ideally, about five parts of the human diet would consist of whole grains, beans, seeds, and other tough plant fibers; two parts, local vegetables; and up to one part, animal food. The optimum ratio of plant to animal food is about seven to one.

It is to our advantage to eat primarily plant foods. Our intestines are long and convoluted compared with those of carnivorous (meat-eating) animals. The digestive systems of carnivorous animals promote rapid food transit; as a result, the toxic byproducts of decaying animal flesh are less likely to accumulate. But in our case, a diet high in animal foods transits through our digestive systems much more slowly, allowing toxins to accumulate throughout the body. Ultimately, this results in a variety of disorders, including cancer. Moreover, studies have shown that as we increase our consumption of animal foods, our intake of beneficial fiber begins to go down. Fiber is found naturally in whole grains, beans, vegetables, and other plant foods, and reduces the risk of digestive disorders, including cancer of the colon.

PREVENTIVE DIETS ARE TRADITIONALLY BASED

The rising incidence of cancer and other chronic diseases parallels the shift away from the traditional patterns of eating and toward the modern diet high in saturated fat, sugar, and refined foods. This shift has taken place mostly during the twentieth century, and (despite the recent impact of the natural food movement) has accelerated since World War II. At the same time, cancer rates have also increased. For example, when I came to this country in the early 1950s, about one out of seven Americans was expected to develop cancer. Today, the National Cancer Institute estimates that one out of three will eventually develop it.

Why the Modern Diet Contributes to Disease

Below we look at features of the modern, non-traditionally-based diet that have contributed to the rise of cancer and other chronic illnesses.

Too Much Fat

During the twentieth century, meat and other animal products became the mainstay of the modern diet. (Refer to Figure 1.1, following.) These foods are high in saturated fat and cholesterol, and are linked with increasing rates of several leading forms of cancer, including cancer of the colon. Moreover, as intake of animal food increases, intake of beneficial fiber normally decreases. A high intake of fiber, such as that found in whole grains, beans, and fresh vegetables, is associated with lower rates of certain cancers, especially those of the large intestine.

At present, about 42 percent of the average U.S. diet is composed of fat, while in rural Mexico, among the Tarahumara, a native people known for their longevity as well as their freedom from cancer and de-

**Figure 1.1   Per Capita Consumption of
Meat, Fish, and Poultry in the U.S.
1900–1980**

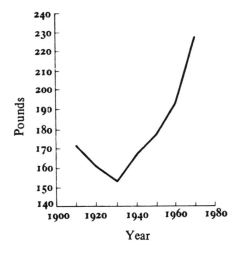

Source: The National Cancer Institute,
Diet, Nutrition and Cancer Program,
Status Report. July, 1976.

generative sicknesses, the amount is only about 12 percent. Approximately 15 percent of the standard macrobiotic diet consists of fat, mostly in the form of vegetable oil.

The American Cancer Society reported in January 1987 that one out of ten American women will develop breast cancer—an all-time high. A decade before, the chances of getting breast cancer were one in thirteen. In an interview published in the *Boston Globe*, Dr. Virgil Loeb, president of the society, stated that fat in the diet and obesity were both involved in the development of the disease.

The relationship between cancer of the colon—a leading killer—and high-fat diets (which raise cholesterol levels) has been known for some time. In December 1986, the *New England Journal of Medicine* added to the evidence with a report on a study in which men with high cholesterol levels were found to be about 60 percent more likely to develop colon cancer than were those with normal cholesterol levels. A similar study found a relationship between high cholesterol and colon polyps that often turn cancerous. Meat, eggs, dairy foods, and other animal products are the chief sources of saturated fat and cholesterol in the modern diet.

When we consider these studies along with research conducted more than ten years ago by Harvard Medical School, it becomes clear that the macrobiotic diet has tremendous potential in the prevention of cancer. The Harvard researchers tested more than 200 macrobiotic people in the Boston area and found that they had cholesterol levels that were far below the normally high averages in the United States.

With new evidence linking high cholesterol with cancer of the colon, it seems reasonable to state that people who eat a naturally balanced diet of whole grains, beans, and fresh vegetables, with little or no animal food, rarely, if ever, develop colon cancer.

Moreover, a naturally balanced diet in the direction of macrobiotics may also offer the best hope of preventing breast cancer, by lowering the overall intake of fat and reducing the tendency toward obesity.

Too Many Simple Sugars

Traditional diets were based on complex carbohydrates, such as whole cereal grains, fresh local vegetables, beans, seasonal fruits, and other foods. A complex carbohydrate (or "complex sugar") is made up of many molecules of simple sugar bound together in a long chain. In their natural form, complex carbohydrates, including fiber, exist together with a balanced mix of proteins, vitamins, and minerals.

Unfortunately, we have shifted from these naturally balanced carbohydrates to simple sugars such as refined cane or beet sugar, fructose, and corn syrup. (Refer to Figure 1.2, following.) The average American con-

**Figure 1.2   Per Capita Refined Sugar Consumption
in the U.S., 1860–1980**

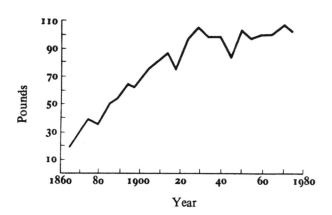

Source: The National Cancer Institute,
Diet, Nutrition and Cancer Program,
Status Report. July, 1976.

sumes more than 100 pounds of refined sugar every year! When the consumption of sugar was much lower, so were incidences of cancer and heart disease.

In the normal digestive process, complex sugars are metabolized gradually and at a nearly even rate by various enzymes in the mouth, stomach, pancreas, and intestines. Complex sugars enter the bloodstream slowly after being broken down into smaller units. During this process, the normal acid-alkaline balance of the blood is not disturbed; the blood remains slightly alkaline.

In contrast, simple sugars are metabolized quickly, enter the bloodstream quickly, and cause the blood to become overacidic. To compensate for this, the pancreas secretes insulin, a substance that promotes the removal of excess sugar from the blood and makes it easier for the sugar to enter the cells of the body. Diabetes can be characterized by the failure of the pancreas to produce enough insulin to neutralize excess blood sugar following years of extreme dietary consumption.

The liver absorbs glucose (the end product of all sugar metabolism) from the blood and stores it, in the form of glycogen, until it is needed by the body. Then it is again changed into glucose. When the liver exceeds its storage capacity of about 50 grams, glucose may be released into the bloodstream in the form of fatty acid. This fatty acid is stored first in the more inactive places of the body, such as the buttocks, thighs, and midsection. Then if cane sugar, fruit sugar, and other simple sugars continue to be eaten, fatty acid becomes attracted to internal organs such as the heart, liver, and kidneys, which gradually become encased in a layer of fat and mucus.

This accumulation can also penetrate the inner tissues, weakening the normal functioning of the organs and causing their eventual blockage, as in the case of atherosclerosis. This buildup of fat set in motion by over-consumption of refined sugar can also lead to various forms of cancer, including tumors of the breast, colon, and reproductive organs. Other forms of degeneration may occur when the body's internal supply of minerals is mobilized to offset the debilitating effects of simple sugar consumption. For example, calcium from the teeth may be depleted to balance the excessive intake of candy, soft drinks, and sugary desserts.

In order to prevent these degenerative effects, it is best to minimize or avoid eating refined carbohydrates, dairy foods, and fruits (which contain the naturally occurring sugars lactose and fructose). Instead, eat complex carbohydrates, in the forms found in grains, beans and bean products, vegetables, and sea-vegetables.

Too Many Refined Foods

A typical modern diet, high in white bread, cane sugar, white rice, and refined table salt, easily leads to nutritional imbalance and deficiency. According to the National Academy of Sciences, about 55 percent of the food consumed in the United States has been refined or processed to some degree before reaching the consumer.

This refining or processing leads to nutrient loss. For example, when whole wheat flour is milled into white flour, much of the germ (embryo), bran, and surface endosperm are removed. As a result, the flour loses most of its energy and vitality as well as its natural oils and nutrients. Though a few of the vitamins and minerals are artificially returned in enriching, the resulting quality is not the same. Refer to Table 1.1, following, which shows the typical loss of nutrients in producing white flour.

Vitamin pills and other nutritional supplements have become popular in recent years to offset the deficiencies, and in extreme cases, deficiency diseases, caused by modern food processing. In essence, the vitamins and minerals taken out of whole foods are sold back to the consumer in capsule form. When taken in this unnatural way to supplement our regular food, vitamin pills produce a chaotic effect on the body's metabolism.

For hundreds of thousands of years, humanity has taken vitamins in whole form. This practice is respected by the macrobiotic dietary approach and is beginning to find acceptance in some scientific circles. For example, in *Diet, Nutrition and Cancer*, the National Academy of Sciences concluded, "Adverse effects result, at least partly, from the availability (and overuse) of vitamin and mineral supplements. Certain vitamins and

Table 1.1 Nutrients Lost in Refining Wheat Flour

Nutrient	Loss (percent)
Thiamine (B₁)	77.1
Riboflavin (B₂)	80.0
Niacin	80.8
Vitamin B₆	71.8
Pantothenic acid	50.0
Vitamin E	86.3
Calcium	60.0
Phosphorus	70.9
Magnesium	84.7
Potassium	77.0
Sodium	78.3
Chromium	40.0
Manganese	85.8
Iron	75.6
Cobalt	88.5
Copper	67.9
Zinc	77.7
Selenium	15.9
Molybdenum	48.0

Source: Henry A. Schroeder, "Losses of Vitamins and Trace Minerals Resulting from Processing and Preservation of Foods" *American Journal of Clinical Nutrition,* 24:562-573, 1971.

most of the minerals are known to be toxic above certain levels."

Commenting on the role of certain vitamins in cancer prevention, and the need to take these substances in their whole form, the National Academy of Sciences stated:

> It is important to include fruits, vegetables, and whole grains in the daily diet. Various components of these foods, including some vitamins and other substances, have been shown to be of potential benefit in the prevention of cancer. However, the importance of these compounds does not justify the use of supplements to increase their intake. Because of the unknown and potentially toxic effects of supplements, this recommendation applies to foods as sources of nutrients—not to dietary supplements of individual nutrients.

A balanced whole foods diet contains various kinds of whole cereal grains, beans and bean products, vegetables, sea-vegetables, fruits, seeds and nuts, and occasional animal food if desired. It uses good-quality unrefined vegetable oil for cooking and naturally processed sea salt.

(Sea salt, the traditional type of salt used in macrobiotic cooking, retains all the natural mineral compounds and trace elements found in the sea.) Most important, a balanced whole foods diet supplies all essential nutrients in natural form.

Too Many Chemicals

Traditional cancer prevention diets were basically natural and organic. The use of artificial chemicals in the human diet began in the twentieth century and corresponds to the rise of cancer and other degenerative diseases. Today, more than 3,000 additives are used to color, flavor, preserve, and extend the shelf life of foods, including fresh fruits and vegetables. A variety of herbicides, pesticides, and fertilizers are routinely used on crops. Commercial livestock and poultry are fed artificial growth hormones and antibiotics, and their feed is usually contaminated with chemicals.

Chemical additives have been linked to a variety of disorders, including hyperactivity, allergies, hormone imbalances, and cancer.

Foods grown in mineral-poor soil that has been depleted by chemical fertilizers, pesticides, and other sprays lose vitamins and minerals that are important for good nutrition. Scientific tests show that organic fruits and vegetables, which are grown in naturally enriched soil without the use of any chemicals, contain up to three times more minerals and trace elements. Refer to Table 1.2, following, which shows the amounts of minerals contained in organic and inorganic vegetables.

PREVENTIVE DIETS ARE MODERATELY BALANCED

Cancer prevention diets, both traditional and modern, are the natural outcome of a way of life that is in harmony with nature. In macrobiotics, we use the terms *yin* and *yang* to describe the workings of natural law. They represent the two most basic forces in the universe: yin represents centrifugal, expanding, or upward force or movement; and yang, centripetal, contracting, or downward force or movement.

Since everything in the universe is in motion, yin and yang are present everywhere. However, some things have a more yin, or expansive tendency, and others a more yang or contractive nature. All things come and go, appear and disappear, move and change because of these two primary forces.

The items on the following lists are arranged in descending order from most yang to most yin. The more balanced foods in the center column are generally recommended for consumption in temperate climates, while those in the strong yang and strong yin columns are generally not recom-

Table 1.2 Minerals in Organic and Inorganic Vegetables

	Percentage of dry weight		Mill equivalents per 100 grams dry weight				Trace elements parts per million dry matter				
	Total ash or mineral matter	Phos-pho-rous	Cal-cium	Mag-nesi-um	Potas-sium	Sodi-um	Bo-ron	Man-ganese	Iron	Cop-per	Co-balt
Snap Beans											
Organic	10.45	0.36	40.5	60.0	99.7	8.6	73	60	227	69.0	0.26
Inorganic	4.04	0.22	15.5	14.8	29.1	0.0	10	2	10	3.0	0.00
Cabbage											
Organic	10.38	0.38	60.0	43.6	148.3	20.4	42	13	94	48.0	0.15
Inorganic	6.12	0.18	17.5	13.6	33.7	0.8	7	2	20	0.4	0.00
Lettuce											
Organic	24.48	0.43	71.0	49.3	176.5	12.2	37	169	516	60.0	0.19
Inorganic	7.01	0.22	16.0	13.1	53.7	0.0	6	1	9	3.0	0.00
Tomatoes											
Organic	14.20	0.35	23.0	59.2	148.3	6.5	36	68	1,938	53.0	0.63
Inorganic	6.07	0.16	4.5	4.5	58.8	0.0	3	1	1	0.0	0.00
Spinach											
Organic	28.56	0.52	96.0	203.9	237.0	69.5	88	117	1,584	32.0	0.25
Inorganic	12.38	0.27	47.5	46.9	84.6	0.8	12	1	19	0.3	0.20

Information from "Variations in Mineral Content in Vegetables," Firman E. Baer Report, Rutgers University, 1984. From *Macrobiotic Diet: Balancing Your Eating in Harmony with the Changing Environment and Personal Needs,* By Michio and Aveline Kushi, edited by Alex Jack, Japan Publications, 1985, p. 68.

mended as a part of a preventive lifestyle. Certain items within the centrally-balanced column, such as sea salt and other seasonings, condiments, white-meat fish, seasonal fruits, oils, and concentrated sweeteners, are best used in small amounts only or consumed occasionally. Drugs and medications are included in the lists because, like foods, they are taken into the body.

Foods, like everything else, can be classified into yin and yang categories. In general, animal foods, including meat, eggs, poultry, and hard cheeses, exert a more contractive effect on the body and are rich in hemoglobin, sodium, and other mineral salts. Their quality is generally more yang. Vegetable foods are for the most part more expanded. They exert a relatively relaxing or cooling effect on the body; are rich in chlorophyll, water, and potassium; and are considered more yin. Refer to Table 1.3, following, which lists yin, yang, and more balanced foods.

Among vegetables, those grown in the tropics are more extreme than those grown in temperate climates. Mangoes, oranges, and bananas, for

Table 1.3 General Yin (▽) and Yang (△) Classification of Food

Strong Yang Foods	More Balanced Foods	Strong Yin Foods

Refined salt
Eggs
Meat
Hard Cheese
Poultry
Lobster, crab, and
  other shellfish
Red-meat and
blue-skinned fish
	Unrefined white sea salt,
	  miso, tamari soy sauce,
	  and other naturally salty
	  seasonings
	Tekka, gomashio, umeboshi,
	  and other naturally-
	  processed salty
	  condiments
	Low-fat, white-meat fish
	Sea vegetables
	Whole cereal grains
	Beans and bean products
	Root, round, and leafy
	  green vegetables from
	  temperate climates
	Seeds and nuts from
	  temperate climates
	Fruits grown in
	  temperate climates
	Nonaromatic, non-stimulant
	  beverages
	Spring or well water
	Naturally-processed
	  vegetable oils
	Brown rice syrup, barley
	  malt, and other natural
	  grain-based sweeteners
	  (when used moderately)
		White rice, white flour
		Frozen and canned foods
		Tropical fruits and vegetables
		  including those originating
		  in the tropics—e.g.,
		  tomatoes and potatoes
		Milk, cream, yogurt, and ice
		  cream
		Refined oils
		Spices (pepper, curry, nutmeg,
		  etc.)
		Aromatic and stimulant
		  beverages (coffee, black tea,
		  mint tea, etc.)
		Honey, sugar, and refined
		  sweeteners
		Alcohol
		Foods containing chemicals,
		  preservatives, dyes, and
		  pesticides
		Artificial sweeteners
		Drugs (marijuana, cocaine, etc.,
		  with some exceptions)
		Medications (tranquilizers,
		  antibiotics, etc., with some
		  exceptions)

example, are more yin than apples or pears. Leafy expanded vegetables, such as lettuce, Chinese cabbage, and bok choy, are more yin than compact root vegetables such as carrots or burdock root. Refined sugar, extracted from tropical sugarcane, is extremely yin in comparison to sweeteners derived from the complex carbohydrates in grains such as rice and barley.

Like the opposite poles of a magnet, yin and yang attract one another. The more extreme the diet becomes at one end, the more we require opposite extremes to make balance. In this century, rising intakes of meat and poultry (yang foods), for example, have required progressively more powerful forms of yin to make balance.

Sugar, chocolate, tomatoes, coffee, and spices are commonly used today. But, beyond these, many people turn to the frequent consumption of alcohol, or to drugs, which are even more extreme. The foods that macrobiotic eating is based upon—whole grains, beans and their products, fresh local vegetables, sea-vegetables, and others—are more centrally balanced than are extremes such as these. This more centrally balanced way of eating helps people to maintain harmony with the planetary environment while avoiding the extremes that can lead to cancer and other degenerative diseases.

As we have seen, during the twentieth century, people have changed from more balanced patterns of eating to more extreme diets. Rather than incorporating balanced complex carbohydrates, such as those in whole grains and vegetables, the modern diet relies heavily on extremely yin simple sugars. In place of the balanced proteins found in whole grains and beans, our modern way of eating emphasizes extreme animal proteins, including meat, eggs, and poultry. The overintake of these dietary extremes is an underlying cause of the modern epidemic of degenerative diseases, including cancer.

PREVENTIVE DIETS BALANCE CLIMATE AND SEASON

The more balanced foods in the macrobiotic diet—whole grains, beans, fresh local vegetables, and more northern varieties of fruit—are generally the products of the temperate zone. As we have seen, they were the mainstay of traditional diets in these regions until the modern age. The development of the modern diet represents a movement away from these traditional staples toward foods that are more appropriate in the polar or tropical regions.

Today, most Americans, Europeans, Japanese, and Soviets eat large amounts of meat and dairy products suited to a colder, semipolar climate, along with fruits and vegetables native to the tropics, refined sugar and spices from the tropics, and cola beverages, coffee, and other stimulants prepared from tropical ingredients. This way of eating in a temperate zone violates the ecological order and sooner or later leads to physical or mental imbalance.

Modern methods of food preparation, storage, and transportation have also made it harder for us to vary our diet in accordance with the changing seasons. Today, people can eat ice cream and frozen yogurt in the winter and barbecued ribs during the heat of July, and have lost touch with nature and genuine health. These eating patterns have contributed to the rise of degenerative illness.

Adjusting diet to meet seasonal change is an important part of a preventive lifestyle. Those who would like to know more about cooking with the seasons can refer to *The Changing Seasons Macrobiotic Cookbook* (Avery Publishing Group, 1985).

The intake of soft drinks, ice cream, orange juice, chilled beverages, and other extreme yin items is one reason why people in northern regions develop colds and flu so frequently during the autumn and winter. These items cause fewer symptoms during the hot dry weather of summer, but as the weather turns colder (more yin), the body seeks to discharge them.

Discharge can take many forms, including sneezing, coughing, chills and fever, and digestive upsets. When handled properly, symptoms like these can be beneficial. They allow the body to discharge toxins, and indicate that natural immunity is still working. However, aspirin and other medications weaken the body's natural ability to discharge. Excess that would normally come out during a cold goes elsewhere; usually toward the internal organs and lymph glands. This sets the stage for many problems. It can lead to formation of deposits of mucus and fat in and around the organs, tissues, and glands, and eventual deterioration of the body's cells. In order to remain free of these conditions, it is important to eat in harmony with our climate and to vary our diet with the seasons.

As we have seen, modern nutritional studies, such as *Dietary Goals* and *Diet, Nutrition and Cancer,* are pointing in the direction of macrobiotics. Modern science is revealing what macrobiotics has been saying all along: a naturally balanced diet is essential in maintaining health and freedom from cancer and other degenerative diseases.

Chapter Two
PREVENTIVE GUIDELINES

This macrobiotic diet appears to be nutritionally adequate if the mix of foods in the dietary recommendations are followed carefully. There is no apparent evidence of any nutritional deficiencies among current macrobiotic practices. . . . The diet would also be consistent with the recently released dietary guidelines of the National Academy of Sciences and the American Cancer Society in regard to possible reduction of cancer risks.

—*Congressional Subcommittee on Health and Long-Term Care, 1984.*

Over the last decade, many people have gradually become aware of the limits of chemical agriculture and food technology. Recent medical studies show that most of the foods in the macrobiotic diet protect against cancer and other degenerative diseases. In the macrobiotic view, cancer is not an isolated condition, but a disease of the whole body.

MEDICAL FINDINGS ABOUT FOOD

Naturally balanced and naturally prepared foods can substantially reduce the risk of cancer in general. Briefly let us look at the major medical findings as they apply to the basic categories of food in the standard macrobiotic diet.

Whole Grains

A wide variety of studies show that, as a part of a balanced diet, whole grains, which are high in fiber and bran, protect against nearly all forms of cancer. The Senate Select Committee's report *Dietary Goals for the United States*, the Surgeon General's document *Healthy People*, the National Academy of Sciences' report *Diet, Nutrition and Cancer*, and many others call for substantial increases in the daily consumption of whole grains such as brown rice, millet, barley, oats, and whole wheat. Whole cereal grains are eaten daily in the macrobiotic diet.

Soup

Soup or broth can play a powerful role in a healthy diet. A ten-year study completed in 1981 by the National Cancer Center in Japan reported that people who ate miso (fermented soybean paste) soup daily were 33 percent less likely to contract stomach cancer than those who never ate miso soup. The study also found that miso was effective in preventing heart and liver diseases. Regular consumption of miso soup is recommended in the macrobiotic diet.

Vegetables

A wide range of studies have shown that regular intake of cooked vegetables, particularly dark green and dark yellow vegetables such as broccoli, carrots, and cabbage, helps protect against cancer. In Japan, a 1970 laboratory study reported that shiitake mushrooms had a strong antitumor effect and no toxic side effects. These and other fresh vegetables are used regularly in the macrobiotic diet. "The dietary changes now under way appear to be reducing our dependence on foods from animal sources," the National Academy of Sciences reported, looking into the future of the American diet; "It is likely that there will be increasing dependence on vegetable and other plant products for protein supplies. Hence, diets may contain increasing amounts of vegetable products, some of which may be protective against cancer."

Beans and Sea-Vegetables

Medical studies indicate that regular consumption of lentils reduces the risk of cancer. In addition, soybeans, a major source of protein in the macrobiotic diet, have been singled out in laboratory tests as especially effective in reducing the incidence of tumors. The active ingredient in soybeans is called a protease inhibitor. Whole soybeans and soy products, including miso, tamari soy sauce, tofu, tempeh, and natto, are macrobiotic staples.

In addition, several medical studies and case history reports indicate that sea-vegetables can be effective in eliminating tumors. In 1974, in the *Japanese Journal of Experimental Medicine*, scientists stated that several varieties of kombu (a common sea-vegetable eaten in Asia and in macrobiotic diets) were effective in the treatment of tumors. In three of four samples tested in the lab, inhibition rates in mice with implanted cancerous tumors ranged from 89 to 95 percent. The researchers reported: "The tumor underwent complete regression in more than half of the mice of each treated group." Similar experiments, in which mice with leukemia (cancer of the blood) were treated with sea-vegetables, showed promising results.

In 1984, medical researchers at Harvard University reported that a diet containing 5 percent kombu significantly delayed the inducement of breast cancer in experimental animals. Extrapolating these results to human subjects, the investigators concluded, "Seaweed may be an important factor in explaining the low rates of certain cancers in Japan." Japanese women, whose diet normally includes about 5 percent sea-vegetables, have an incidence of breast cancer that is from three to nine times lower than the rate among American women, for whom sea-vegetables are not part of the regular way of eating.

Plants from the sea may also protect against radioactivity. Medical doctors in Nagasaki who helped save their patients on a traditional diet of brown rice, miso soup, and sea-vegetables after the atomic bombing in 1945 attested to this. In addition, scientists at McGill University in Canada reported in the 1960s and 1970s that common edible sea-vegetables contained a substance that selectively combined with radioactive strontium and helped eliminate it naturally from the body. The substance, sodium alginate, was prepared from kombu, kelp, and other brown sea-vegetables found off Atlantic and Pacific coastal waters. "The evaluation of biological activity of different marine algae is important because of their practical significance in preventing absorption of radioactive products of atomic fission as well as in their use of possible natural decontaminators," the researchers concluded in an article in the *Canadian Medical Association Journal*.

MACROBIOTICS AS A PREVENTIVE LIFESTYLE

Macrobiotics offers more than just an orderly way of eating. It encompasses a whole lifestyle that respects human tradition and the order of nature, with the spirit of fostering personal and social well-being and creating a healthy and peaceful world.

We focus on diet because, as we have seen, a properly balanced diet can play a primary role in lowering the risk of cancer and other degenerative illnesses. Let us now examine the outlines of the standard macrobiotic diet. This way of eating, with appropriate modifications for each individual, can serve as the basis for a more healthful and preventive lifestyle.

In contrast to modern dietary habits, macrobiotic eating is based on the following nutritional considerations:

- More complex carbohydrates and fewer simple sugars;
- More good-quality protein from vegetables, and less protein from animal sources;
- Less overall consumption of fat—more unsaturated fat and less saturated fat;
- Adequate consideration of the ideal balance between vitamins, minerals, and other nutritional factors;
- Use of more natural, high-quality, organically grown foods and fewer chemically sprayed or fertilized items;
- Use of more traditionally processed foods and fewer artificially and chemically processed foods;
- A larger intake of foods in their whole form and a smaller intake of refined and partial foods;
- Consumption of foods rich in natural fiber rather than foods that have been devitalized.

The macrobiotic way of eating is similar in orientation to dietary guidelines issued by a number of public health agencies. Some of these are identified below.

- The United States Congress, Senate Select Committee on Nutrition and Human Needs. (Publication: *Dietary Goals for the United States,* 1977);
- The U.S. Surgeon General. *Healthy People: Health Promotion and Disease Prevention* (1979 report);
- The American Heart Association, the American Diabetes Association, the American Society for Clinical Nutrition, and the U.S. Department of Agriculture;

- A panel of the American Association for the Advancement of Science (1981 report);
- The National Academy of Sciences. (The dietary guidelines for cancer prevention issued in the 1982 report *Diet, Nutrition and Cancer*);
- The American Cancer Society. (Dietary guidelines issued in 1984.)

The macrobiotic guidelines have been practiced daily for more than twenty years by hundreds of thousands of people throughout the world, including many families. Moreover, similar dietary practices have been observed traditionally by many cultures for thousands of years.

The guidelines in this chapter are designed for people living in temperate climates. Modifications are required if you live in a tropical or subtropical climate, or in a polar or semipolar region. We also need to adjust our diet when we travel or move to one of these regions. It is also important to flexibly adapt these guidelines to suit every individual's needs and condition. For this reason, it is a good idea to meet with a qualified macrobiotic teacher or to participate in programs such as the Macrobiotic Way of Life Seminar presented by the Kushi Institute in Boston, in order to receive individual guidance. (A schedule of these ongoing programs is available from the Kushi Foundation.)

THE STANDARD MACROBIOTIC DIET

The standard macrobiotic way of eating offers an incredible variety of foods and cooking methods from which to choose. The guidelines that follow are broad and flexible. You can apply them when selecting the highest quality natural foods for yourself and your family. Refer to Figure 2.1, following, which details the standard macrobiotic diet.

Whole Cereal Grains

Whole cereal grains are the staff of life and are an essential part of a healthful preventive way of eating. For people living in temperate climates, whole grains may comprise up to 50 to 60 percent of daily food intake. Below is a list of the standard whole grains and grain products that may be included in the macrobiotic diet.

Brown Rice
Short, medium, and
  long grain brown rice
Genuine brown rice cream
Puffed brown rice
Brown rice flakes

Sweet Brown Rice
Sweet brown rice (grain)
Mochi (pounded sweet
  brown rice)
Sweet brown rice flour products

Barley
Barley grain
Pearl barley (hato mugi)
Pearled barley
Puffed barley
Barley flour products

Whole Wheat
Whole wheat berries
Whole wheat bread
Whole wheat chapatis
Whole wheat noodles and pastas
Whole wheat flakes
Whole wheat bread flour
Whole wheat pastry flour
Whole wheat flour products
    such as crackers, matzos,
    muffins, etc.
Cracked wheat
Couscous
Bulghur
Fu (baked puffed wheat gluten)
Seitan (wheat gluten)

Millet
Millet grain
Millet flour products
Puffed millet

Oats
Whole Oats
Steel-cut oats
Rolled Oats
Oatmeal
Oat flakes
Oat flour products

Corn
Corn on the cob
Corn grits
Cornmeal
Arepas
Corn flour products (bread,
    muffins, etc.)
Puffed corn
Popped corn

Rye
Rye grain
Rye bread
Rye flakes
Rye flour products

Buckwheat
Buckwheat groats (kasha)
Buckwheat noodles and pastas
Buckwheat flour products
    (e.g., pancakes, crepes, etc.)

Cooked whole grains are easier to digest than flour products or cracked or rolled grains. In general, it is better to keep your intake of flour products—or cracked or rolled grains—to less than 15 to 20 percent of your daily whole grain consumption.

Soups

In the macrobiotic way of eating, soups may comprise about 5 percent of each person's daily intake. For most people, that averages out to about one or two cups or small bowls of soup per day, depending on their desires and preferences. Soups provide us with wonderful variety in our daily fare. They can include vegetables, grains, beans, sea-vegetables,

Figure 2.1 The Standard Macrobiotic Diet

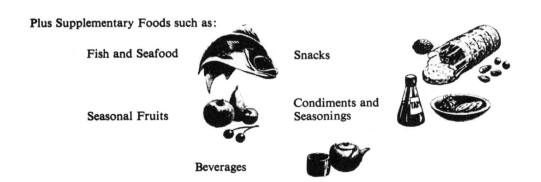

Whole Cereal
Grains 50–60%

Soup
5%

Vegetables
25–30%

Beans and
Sea Vegetables
5–10%

Plus Supplementary Foods such as:

Fish and Seafood   Snacks

Seasonal Fruits   Condiments and
                                    Seasonings

Beverages

noodles or other grain products, bean products like tofu or tempeh, and occasionally, fish or seafood. They can be moderately seasoned with miso, tamari soy sauce, sea salt, umeboshi plum or paste, or (occasionally) ginger.

Soups can be made either thick and rich, or as simple clear broths. Vegetable, grain, or bean stews can also be enjoyed, while a variety of garnishes, such as scallions, parsley, nori sea-vegetable, and croutons, may be used to enhance the appearance and flavor of soups.

Vegetables

Throughout the temperate regions of the world, nature provides us with an incredible variety of local vegetables to choose from. Some of those recommended for regular use are listed below. Roughly one-quarter to one-third (25 to 30 percent) of each person's daily intake can include vegetables. Vegetables can be served in soups—or with grains, beans, or sea-vegetables. They can also be used in the preparation of rice rolls (macro-biotic sushi), served with noodles or pasta, cooked with fish, or served alone.

Acorn squash	Endive
Bok choy	Escarole
Broccoli	Green beans
Burdock root	Green peas
Buttercup squash	Hokkaido pumpkin
Butternut squash	Hubbard squash
Cabbage	Iceberg lettuce
Carrot tops	Jerusalem artichokes
Carrots	Jinenjo
Cauliflower	(Japanese mountain potato)
Celery	Kale
Celery root	Kohlrabi
Chard	Leeks
Chinese cabbage	Lotus root and seeds
Chives	Mushrooms
Collard greens	Mustard greens
Cucumbers	Onions
Daikon	Parsley
Daikon greens	Parsnips
Dandelion greens	Patty pan squash
Dandelion root	Pumpkins

Radishes	Summer squash
Red cabbage	Turnip greens
Romaine lettuce	Turnips
Scallions	Watercress
Shiitake mushrooms	Wax beans

The methods for preparing vegetables that are introduced in this book include boiling, steaming, pressing, sautéing (both waterless and with oil), and pickling. A variety of natural seasonings, including miso, tamari soy sauce, sea salt, and brown rice vinegar or umeboshi vinegar, are recommended in vegetable cookery.

Beans, Peas, and Bean Products

Approximately 5 to 10 percent of your daily food intake may include beans, peas, and bean products. Select from any of the beans, peas, or bean products listed below; you may prepare them in a number of different ways.

Beans and Peas

Azuki beans	Lentils (green and red)
Bean sprouts	Lima beans
Black-eyed peas	Mung beans
Black turtle beans	Navy beans
Black soybeans	Pinto beans
Chick peas (garbanzo beans)	Soybeans
Great Northern beans	Split peas
Kidney beans	Whole dried peas

Bean Products

Dried tofu (soybean curd that has been naturally dried)
Fresh tofu (soybean curd)
Okara (pulp or residue left from making tofu)
Natto (fermented soybeans)
Tempeh (fermented soybeans or combination of soybeans and grains)
Yuba (dried soymilk)

Beans, peas, and bean products are more easily digested when they're cooked with a modest amount of seasonings such as sea salt, miso, or kombu sea-vegetable. They may also be prepared with vegetables, chestnuts, dried apples, or raisins. Occasionally, they may be sweetened with grain sweeteners like barley malt or rice honey. Beans, peas, and bean products may be served in soups and side dishes, or cooked with grains or sea-vegetables.

Sea-Vegetables

Sea-vegetables are both flavorful and healthful, and they may be used daily in cooking. Side dishes made with arame or hiziki can be included in the diet several times per week. Wakame and kombu can be used daily in miso and other soups, in vegetable and bean dishes, or as condiments. Toasted nori is also recommended for regular daily use. Agar-agar can be used from time to time in making a natural jelled dessert known as kanten. (By the way, agar-agar has natural laxative properties.) The sea-vegetables used in macrobiotic cooking are listed below.

Arame	Mekabu
Agar-agar	Nekombu
Dulse	Nori
Hiziki	Sea palm
Irish moss	Wakame
Kombu	

Fish and Seafood

Fish and seafood can be eaten on occasion to supplement the foods discussed above. The amounts eaten can vary, depending upon each person's needs and desires. As a general guideline, however, it is appropriate to eat fish and seafood several times per week as a part of a balanced meal. White-meat varieties are lowest in saturated fat and most easily digested; these are the best for regular use.

Fish (Regular Use)

Carp	Scrod
Cod	Smelt
Flounder	Snapper
Haddock	Sole
Halibut	Trout
Herring	Other white-meat fish

Seafood (Occasional Use)	Infrequent Use
Cherrystone clams	Bluefish
Crab	Salmon
Littleneck clams	Sardines
Lobster	Swordfish
Oysters	Tuna
Shrimp	Other blue-skinned
Small dried fish (iriko)	and red-meat fish

Garnishes are especially important in making sure that meals which contain fish and seafood are well-balanced. Recommended garnishes include: chopped scallions or parsley, grated raw daikon, ginger, radish or horseradish, wasabi (green mustard paste), raw salad, and shredded daikon.

Fruit

Most individuals can enjoy fruit three or four times per week. Locally grown or temperate-climate fruits are preferable; tropical fruits are not recommended for regular use by people in temperate regions. Some of the varieties of fruit for consumption in moderate climates are listed below.

Apples	Peaches
Apricots	Pears
Blackberries	Persimmons
Canteloupe	Plums
Cherries	Raisins
Currants	Raspberries
Grapes	Strawberries
Honeydew melon	Tangerines
Lemons	Watermelon
Mulberries	Wild Berries

Pickles

Pickles can be eaten frequently as a supplement to main dishes. They stimulate appetite and help digestion. Some varieties—such as pickled daikon, or takuan—can be bought prepackaged in natural food stores. Others, such as "quick pickles," can be prepared at home. Certain varieties take just a few hours to prepare, while others require more time.

Many kinds of pickles are fine for regular use, including salt, salt brine, bran, miso, tamari, and umeboshi vinegar. Sauerkraut may also be used, in small amounts, on a regular basis.

Seeds and Nuts

Seeds and nuts can be eaten from time to time as snacks. They can be roasted with or without sea salt, sweetened with barley or rice malt, or seasoned with tamari soy sauce. They can be ground to make spreadable butters. Seeds and nuts can also be shaved and served as a topping, garnish, or ingredient in various dishes, including dessert. The varieties that can be used are listed below.

Nuts (Somewhat Regular Use)
Almonds
Chestnuts
Filberts
Peanuts
Pecans
Pine nuts
Small Spanish nuts
Walnuts

Nuts (Infrequent Use)
Brazil nuts
Cashews
Macadamia nuts
Others

Seeds (Regular Use)
Pumpkin seeds
Sesame seeds (black and tan)
Squash seeds

Seeds (Occasional or Infrequent Use)
Alfalfa seeds
Poppy seeds
Sunflower seeds
Umeboshi plum seeds
Others

Snacks

A variety of natural snacks may be enjoyed from time to time, including those made from whole grains, like cookies, bread, puffed cereals, mochi (pounded sweet brown rice), rice cakes, rice balls, and macrobiotic sushi. Nuts and seeds may also be used as snacks.

Condiments

Condiments can be sprinkled on foods to adjust taste and nutritional value, and to stimulate appetite. A variety of condiments may be used, some daily and others occasionally. They can be used in small amounts on grains, vegetables, and beans; in soups; and sometimes even in desserts. The most frequently used varieties are listed below, along with a few condiments that can be used occasionally.

Condiments (Frequent Use)
Gomashio (roasted sesame seeds and sea salt)
Sea-vegetable powders (with or without roasted sesame seeds)
Tekka (a special condiment made with soybean miso, sesame oil,
    burdock, lotus root, carrots, and ginger)
Umeboshi plums

Condiments (Occasional Use)
Roasted sesame seeds
Roasted and chopped shiso (pickled beefsteak plant) leaves
Shio kombu (kombu cooked with tamari and water)
Green nori flakes
Cooked nori condiment
Cooked miso with scallions or onions
Umeboshi or brown rice vinegar

Condiments can be purchased at the natural food store or made at home and kept in tightly-sealed glass jars or containers. Homemade condiments are fresher than store-bought varieties, and the ingredients can be specially balanced to suit your needs. Homemade varieties include gomashio (black or tan), sea-vegetable powders (with or without roasted sesame seeds), cooked nori condiment, shio kombu, and others. Recipes for preparing these condiments are presented in Chapter Four.

Seasonings

A variety of seasonings can be used when you're cooking macrobiotically. It is best to avoid strong spicy seasonings such as curry, hot pepper, and others, and to use only mild seasonings that have been naturally processed from vegetable products or natural sea salt. Many of these seasonings have been in use for years as a part of traditional diets in the temperate climates of North America, Europe, and the Far East. A list of such seasonings is presented below.

Unrefined sea salt
Tamari soy sauce (fermented soybean and grain sauce)
Miso (fermented soybean and grain paste; e.g., rice [kome miso], barley
    [mugi miso], soybean [hatcho miso], sesame, and other misos)
Brown rice and umeboshi vinegar
Barley malt and rice syrup

Grated daikon, radish, and ginger
Umeboshi plum and paste
Lemon, tangerine, and orange juice
Green and yellow mustard paste
Sesame, corn, safflower, mustard seed, and olive oil
Mirin (fermented sweet brown rice sweetener)
Amasake (fermented sweet brown rice beverage)
Other traditional natural seasonings

Garnishes

A variety of garnishes can be used to create balance among dishes and facilitate digestion. The use of garnishes depends upon the needs and desires of each person. The garnishes that can be used include the ones listed below.

Grated daikon (for fish, mochi, noodles, and other dishes)
Grated radish (use like grated daikon)
Grated horseradish (use mostly for fish and seafood)
Chopped scallions (for noodles, fish and seafood, fried rice, grain or
    bean soups, etc.)
Parsley
Lemon, tangerine, and orange slices (mainly for fish and seafood)

Desserts

A variety of natural desserts may be eaten from time to time. It is best to have these at the end of the main meal. Desserts can be made from azuki beans (sweetened with grain syrup, chestnuts, squash, or raisins); cooked or dried fruit; agar-agar (natural sea-vegetable gelatin); grains (e.g., rice pudding, couscous cake, Indian pudding, etc.); and flour products (such as cookies, cakes, pies, muffins, etc.) prepared with fruit or grain sweeteners.

Beverages

A variety of beverages may be consumed daily or occasionally. Amounts can vary according to each person's needs and the weather conditions. The beverages listed below can be used to comfortably satisfy the desire for liquid.

Bancha twig and stem tea
Roasted brown rice or barley tea

Cereal grain coffee
Spring or well water
Amasake
Dandelion tea
Soybean milk (prepared with kombu)
Sweet vegetable drink
Kombu tea
Lotus root tea
Mu tea
Other traditional non-stimulant and nonaromatic natural herbal
    beverages
Sake (rice wine, without chemicals or sugar)
Beer (natural, high-quality varieties)
Apple, grape, and apricot juice
Apple cider
Carrot, celery, and other vegetable juices

Additional Foods

In some cases, the standard macrobiotic diet can be temporarily modified
to include other foods. Modifications can be made according to individual requirements and necessity, though within usual practice, additional
foods are not necessary for the maintenance of health and well-being.

For Those with Cancer or Serious Illness

The dietary guidelines presented in this chapter are generally for persons
in normally good health who wish to lower their risk of cancer or other
serious illness. However, not all of the foods listed in this section, or in
the recipes in Chapter Four, are recommended for those with cancer or
other serious illnesses. The general guidelines in this book are meant to
be modified and adapted to meet the needs of each individual. Persons
with cancer or another serious illness are advised to attend programs
such as the Macrobiotic Way of Life Seminar presented by the Kushi Institute in Boston, for personal instruction. At the same time, general dietary guidelines for those with cancer are presented in *The Cancer Prevention Diet*, by Michio Kushi with Alex Jack, St. Martin's Press, 1983. We
recommend reviewing this book when applying the guidelines for food
selection and cooking presented here.

SUGGESTIONS FOR HEALTHY LIVING

Together with eating well, there are a number of practices that we recommend for a healthier and more natural life. Keeping physically active and using natural cooking utensils, fabrics, and materials in the home are especially recommended. In the past, people lived more closely with nature and ate a more balanced, natural diet. With each generation, we have gotten further and further from our roots in nature, and have experienced a corresponding increase in cancer and other chronic illnesses. The suggestions presented below complement a balanced natural diet and can help everyone enjoy more satisfying and harmonious living.

- Greet everyone and everything with gratitude, particularly offering thanks before and after each meal. Encourage others to give thanks for their food and their natural environment.
- Live each day happily, without being worried about your health. Keep active mentally and physically. Sing every day and encourage others to join with you.
- Try to get to bed before midnight and get up early in the morning.
- Try not to wear synthetic clothing or woolen articles directly against your skin. Wear cotton instead. Keep jewelry and accessories simple, natural, and graceful.
- If you are able, go outdoors in simple clothing every day. When the weather permits, walk barefoot on the grass, soil, or beach. Go on regular outings, especially to beautiful natural areas.
- Keep your home clean and orderly. Make your kitchen, bathroom, bedrooms, and living rooms shiny and clean. Keep the atmosphere of your home bright and cheerful.
- Maintain an active correspondence. Express love and appreciation to your parents, husband or wife, children, brothers, sisters, relatives, friends, and associates.
- Try not to take long hot baths or showers unless you have been consuming too much salt or animal food.
- Every morning or every night, scrub your whole body with a hot, moist towel until your circulation becomes active. When a complete body scrub is not convenient, at least do your hands, feet, fingers, and toes.
- Use natural cosmetics, soaps, shampoos, and body care products. Brush your teeth with natural preparations or sea salt.
- Keep as active as you can. Daily activities such as cooking, scrubbing floors, cleaning windows, and washing clothes, are excellent forms of exercise. You may also try systematic exercise programs such as yoga, martial arts, aerobics, or sports.
- Try to minimize time spent in front of the television. Color television,

especially, emits radiation that can be physically draining. Turn the TV off during mealtimes. Balance TV-watching with more productive activities.

- Switch from electric to gas cooking at the earliest opportunity. Also, avoid microwave cooking.
- Heating pads, electric blankets, portable radios with earphones, and other electric devices can disrupt the body's natural flow of energy. They are not recommended for regular use.
- Put many green plants in your living room, bedroom, and throughout the house to freshen and enrich the air.

The way in which we eat can be just as important as our choice of foods. It is best to eat regular meals. Be sure to include a whole grain dish at each meal (the word "meal" actually means "crushed whole grain"). The amount of food you eat depends on your needs. But it is always best to keep snacking moderate, so that it doesn't replace meals. Tea and other beverages, however, can be enjoyed throughout the day as desired. Chewing is also important; try to chew each mouthful of food until it becomes liquid. You can eat whenever you feel hungry, but try to avoid eating before bedtime, preferably for three hours, except in unusual circumstances. Finally, learn to appreciate your foods and the health-giving properties they contain. Let your gratitude overflow to include nature, the universe, and all of the people who live on this wonderful planet.

Chapter Three

GETTING STARTED

Over the last twenty years, hundreds of thousands of people in the United States, Canada, Europe, Latin America, the Middle East, Australia, and the Far East have adopted the macrobiotic way of eating and have found it nourishing, satisfying, and delicious. Most people find that soon after changing their diet to focus on whole unprocessed foods, their natural sense of taste returns. After years of eating refined foods and artificially flavored products, our taste buds begin to atrophy and we forget the rich flavors, subtle aromas, and variety of textures offered by whole natural foods. Changing to a natural diet ultimately results not only in improved health but also in recovery of our appetite for life itself.

Changing from the modern diet to a naturally balanced way of eating requires some preparation. In this chapter we focus on how you can get started.

In making the transition from a refined modern diet, it is important to proceed gradually and not try to make the change all at once. Meat and poultry are relatively easy to give up, and most people discover they have little or no desire to consume them after a few weeks. However, if cravings occur, seitan (wheat meat) or tempeh (soy meat) may be consumed frequently in soups, in stews, and with vegetables. When prepared with a whole wheat gravy and served with onions, seitan looks and tastes surprisingly like roast beef. Tempeh often helps diminish the craving for chicken and poultry. Both tofu and tempeh are rich in protein and contain no cholesterol or saturated fat.

In giving up sugar and artificial sweeteners, a steady transition to natural grain sweeteners such as rice syrup and barley malt can be made. It is better to avoid using honey and maple syrup if possible, as these simple sugars can disturb the body's use of energy.

Cravings for sweets are often due to low blood sugar, or hypoglycemia. This condition is very prevalent today; some macrobiotic educators estimate that as many as 60 percent of American adults experience it to one degree or another. A person with hypoglycemia often has strong cravings for sweets, together with mood swings that include depression and anxiety. These symptoms often become acute in the afternoon or evening.

A main cause of hypoglycemia is the overconsumption of foods such as chicken, cheese, eggs, and shellfish. These can make the pancreas become hard and tight, and inhibit its secretion of glucagon, the hormone that causes blood sugar to rise. Avoiding these foods and eating more complex carbohydrates helps solve the problem. Many complex carbohydrate foods have a naturally sweet flavor, and this taste can be emphasized in daily cooking.

At the same time, many people have discovered that hypoglycemia can be relieved fairly quickly by drinking one or two cupfuls of sweet vegetable broth daily. This special drink is made from carrots, cabbage, squash, and onions. To prepare it, finely cut equal amounts of each vegetable. Place the sliced vegetables in a pot and add four times as much water. Bring to a boil, turn the flame to low, and simmer for about 10 minutes. Then, pour the liquid through a fine mesh strainer into a large glass jar. The strained liquid—or "sweet vegetable drink"—can be stored for several days in the refrigerator. One or two cups can be taken daily or several times per week (depending on your condition) until the symptoms of hypoglycemia begin to diminish. To serve sweet vegetable drink, heat it in a saucepan until it is warm, or allow it to sit outside the refrigerator until it reaches room temperature.

All of us have an attachment to the foods on which we were raised. Dairy products were typically the original food of infants and children for several generations of mothers who avoided breastfeeding. It may take a while for modern people, including those who are otherwise nutritionally aware, to overcome an unconscious dependency on dairy products. Products such as amasake and mochi provide an excellent alternative to dairy products, as do tofu and other soybean products. In the natural food kitchen, a wide variety of foods having a taste and texture similar to that of dairy products can be prepared for those whose diets are in transition. Many of these foods are introduced in this book.

In the sections that follow, we present guidelines on learning to cook, shopping for the best ingredients, equipping your kitchen, and preparing food for cooking. These recommendations are designed to make the transition to healthful eating as quick and problem-free as possible.

LEARNING TO COOK

Macrobiotic cooking is quick and simple once a few basic techniques are mastered. Before you learn the basics, however, such as how to use a pressure cooker, wash and cut vegetables, and soak items like shiitake mushrooms and sea-vegetables, it is easy to make mistakes. This is especially true in the beginning when many of the foods and cooking methods are new and unfamiliar. However, like any other skill, you will develop proficiency once you become familiar with the ingredients and methods used in macrobiotic cooking.

Recipes and cookbooks are of course helpful, but the best way to learn about macrobiotic cooking is to attend classes where you can actually see the foods prepared and can taste them. Most introductory macrobiotic cooking classes are presented in a series of six to eight sessions, and will show you how to do important things like wash and soak foods, cut vegetables, purée miso for soup, and combine ingredients in complete meals. Advice on menu planning, setting up your kitchen, and shopping for high quality foods is usually provided as well.

Weekly dinners—which many macrobiotic centers sponsor—are also helpful, as they offer you the chance to see and taste a balanced meal and to talk to other people about macrobiotics in a relaxed and supportive setting.

Until you have actually tasted the full range of macrobiotically prepared foods and seen how they are made, you may not fully appreciate the depth and scope of the possibilities that a more natural way of eating offers, or have a standard against which to measure your own cooking. Cooking is the supreme art, and cookbooks such as this one can only provide general guidance.

Once you have mastered the techniques used daily in macrobiotic cooking, and are able to prepare important basic dishes like pressure-cooked rice, miso soup, steamed or sautéed vegetables, and bean and sea-vegetable side dishes, then you can improvise and experiment on your own and ultimately develop your own unique style with your intuitive sense of balance as your guide.

EQUIPPING YOUR KITCHEN

Before you actually get started in the kitchen, it might be worthwhile to take a brief inventory of your cooking utensils. High-quality cookware can make the difference between a delicious meal and an average one, and can enhance or detract from the natural quality of the foods you prepare. Below are some of the most essential items used in macrobiotic cooking.

Pressure Cooker. A stainless steel pressure cooker is an important utensil for preparing brown rice and other whole grains. A five-liter cooker is usually sufficient for up to six people. There are many fine models to choose from. Ask the salesperson in your natural food store for suggestions on the right model for your needs.

Cookware. Stainless steel cookware is recommended for everyday use. Skillets made from cast iron are also fine for occasional use in sautéing and deep frying. Aluminum, along with teflon and other non-stick coated cookware, is not recommended if you wish to achieve optimum health. Aluminum is absorbed into food, while non-stick or plastic coatings are easily chipped, and minute particles from the surface can get into the food.

Cooking Utensils. Wooden utensils are fairly inexpensive and are made from a material that is harmonious with our everyday needs. Start with basic items such as soup ladles, bamboo rice paddles, a roasting paddle, spoons of various sizes, and cooking chopsticks. Metal tableware is fine if you prefer it, although many people like to use chopsticks and ceramic or wooden spoons, since they prefer the natural feel of wood or clay.

Knives. A high-grade stainless or carbon steel knife is recommended for efficient cutting. Keep your knife properly sharpened, as this can make the difference between smooth and quick cutting and spending unnecessary time in the kitchen. Electric knives and food processors are generally not recommended, as the use of electricity disrupts the natural balance and energy of food.

Cutting Boards. A high-quality wooden cutting board is helpful for cutting vegetables and other foods. You may want to purchase two cutting boards: a larger one for vegetable foods, and a smaller one for fish and seafood.

Flame Deflectors. Flame deflectors are metal pads that are placed under pressure cookers and other pots to distribute heat evenly and prevent burning. Metal flame deflectors are available at variety stores as well as natural food stores.

Natural Bristle Brushes. Small brushes with natural bristles are recommended for cleaning vegetables. They are especially good for scrubbing roots like carrots and burdock, and are available in natural food stores and kitchen specialty shops.

Containers. Glass, ceramic, or wood containers are recommended for storing dried foods. Unlike plastic or metal, they do not change the smell or taste of foods. These containers and jars come in many shapes and sizes, and can be purchased as needed.

Tamari Dispenser. These specially made small glass bottles are used to store tamari soy sauce for handy use. The dispensers make it easy to control the flow of tamari when you add it during cooking.

Strainers and Colanders. A wire mesh strainer or colander is useful for washing and rinsing foods. Large mesh strainers are appropriate for most items, while fine mesh varieties are better for smaller grains and seeds. A bamboo tea strainer is also very useful when straining tea into cups. These items are available at many natural food stores.

Graters. Of the several types of graters available, the most useful is a flat metal vegetable grater. It is very convenient for grating daikon, ginger root, and other vegetables. Other types of graters can also be useful in preparing dishes like sauerkraut or in making salads.

Suribachi. These small Japanese grinding bowls are made of clay and are useful in making gomashio and other condiments, as well as in making sauces, dips, and salad dressings. They are also helpful when purée-ing foods. They come with a small wooden pestle known as a surikogi, and are available in natural food stores.

Pickle Press. This plastic utensil is very useful when preparing quick pickles and pressed salads. Pickle presses are available at many natural food stores. If you can't locate one, you can make pressed salads by placing the cut vegetables in a bowl, putting a plate or saucer on top, and adding a rock or weight of some sort to apply pressure.

Bamboo Sushi Mats. These flexible mats are made from thin strips of bamboo that are connected with string. They are handy to use when you're making macrobiotic sushi or covering dishes of leftovers. It is a good idea to purchase several.

Steamers. The most popular steamers are the collapsible stainless steel variety that fits inside cooking pots, and the bamboo type consisting of several layers that are stacked on a steaming pot of water. Steamers are handy for warming leftovers and (of course) for steaming greens and other foods.

Sharpening Stones. Keeping your vegetable knives properly sharpened makes cooking more enjoyable. The stones for sharpening knives are available at most hardware, natural food, and kitchen specialty shops. When you purchase your knife, ask the salesperson for sharpening instructions.

BASIC SHOPPING LIST

When you buy natural foods, it is important to select from among the highest-quality natural and organic products. Selecting a store that maintains high standards of quality is therefore essential. This is especially important when shopping for essential items such as grains, beans, sea-vegetables, miso, tamari, sea salt, oils, umeboshi (pickled salt plums), seeds, noodles, and breads.

It is best to purchase organic vegetables, but in some cases it may not be possible. If you have difficulty locating organic produce and you have the space, think about starting your own vegetable garden. Organic seeds are available by mail from several seed companies in North America. When necessary, your organic staples can be supplemented with nonorganic produce from local markets. Nonorganic produce should be thoroughly washed and properly cooked to reduce potentially toxic residues.

You may choose to stock your pantry with new foods gradually or all at once. Embarking on a new way of cooking and eating can be fun and exciting. There are natural and macrobiotic food stores in most cities and towns in the United States where you can shop. Several larger distributors have mail order catalogs if you have trouble finding certain items.

Foods can be purchased in small quantities to suit individual or family needs or in larger bulk quantities at reduced prices. Below is a list of staple items that you may want to stock in your kitchen as you begin. As you purchase them, these items can be stored in glass, ceramic, or wooden containers.

Grains. Brown rice (short grain is suitable for four-season climates, while for warmer climates you may also want to use medium grain), barley, pearl barley (sometimes sold under the name *hato mugi*), millet, sweet brown rice, rolled oats, whole oats, wheat berries, kasha (buckwheat), fresh corn in season, and whole rye. Cracked or partially refined grains may be purchased for occasional use, and include bulghur, cracked wheat, and couscous.

Noodles. Whole wheat noodles, (including udon and somen); soba (buckwheat noodles); whole wheat pasta and spaghetti; whole wheat, rice, and buckwheat ramen.

Beans. Azuki beans, lentils, chickpeas, black soybeans, soybeans, black turtle beans, kidney beans, pinto beans, navy beans, Great Northern beans, split peas, whole dried peas, and Lima beans.

Sea-Vegetables. Arame, hiziki, nori, kombu, wakame, dulse, sea palm, and agar-agar.

Condiments and Seasonings. Barley miso, hatcho miso, tamari soy sauce, umeboshi plums, umeboshi paste, umeboshi vinegar, brown rice vinegar, ginger root, barley malt, rice syrup, mirin (a sweet rice cooking wine), and sea salt.

Beverages. Bancha tea, roasted barley tea, and cereal grain coffee.

Seeds and Nuts. Sesame seeds (black and tan), sunflower, and pumpkin seeds. Dried chestnuts, walnuts, almonds, and roasted peanuts.

Flour and Flour Products. Whole wheat bread and pastry flour, buckwheat and corn flour, and cornmeal. Store-bought whole wheat, sour-dough, or rice bread can be used occasionally.

Dried Fruits. Raisins, apples, apricots, currants, cherries, peaches, and pears.

Oils. Unrefined dark sesame oil, light sesame oil, and corn oil.

Others. Special items you might wish to stock include kuzu, arrow-root flour, dried tofu, mochi, amasake, shiitake mushrooms (dried Japanese mushrooms), snacks (rice cakes, puffed cereals, popping corn, etc.), dried daikon, fu, fresh tofu, tempeh, and dried lotus seeds (both white and red), among others.

Perishable items such as fresh vegetables, fresh fruits and tofu can be purchased as needed and stored in the refrigerator when necessary.

IN THE KITCHEN

With your cupboards and refrigerator stocked with high-quality natural foods, you are now ready to try your hand at healthful cooking.

Before you actually begin, it is important to be well prepared. Proper preparation saves time and energy, and gives you more freedom to be creative and apply your natural intuition and sense of balance. We would like to recommend the following practices as you begin cooking:

- Select your materials wisely from organic products naturally grown, in season, and from the climate or region in which you live.
- Try to use whole natural foods that are fresh until the time they are cooked.
- When cutting vegetables or other foods, do them individually and place each separately; avoid mixing vegetables until you begin to cook them. Also, wipe your cutting board clean after cutting each vegetable.
- Try to cut your vegetables as elegantly and gracefully as possible so that each cut is evenly balanced.
- As much as possible, allow the flavors of your foods to mingle during the natural process of cooking.
- Use seasonings moderately. Unrefined sea salt, cold-pressed vegetable oils, natural grain sweeteners, whole grain vinegar, and other recommended seasonings can be used to enhance the natural flavor of food. It is best if the seasoning is kept mild.
- Strong spicy seasonings are usually not appropriate in temperate climates.
- Use the best quality of water for cooking and drinking—clean well, spring, or mountain stream water. City water can be used for washing your foods and utensils. Avoid distilled water.

- Make your dishes more appealing by presenting them beautifully and elegantly. The natural colors of foods can be harmonized through cooking to create colorful and attractive dishes.
- Keep your kitchen and dining area clean and orderly. Keep the atmosphere of your dining area quiet and calm, and maintain a peaceful, loving, and joyful state of mind while cooking and eating.

COOKING FOOD

Proper cooking brings out and enhances the flavor of food, stimulates the appetite, and balances our condition with nature and the environment. By varying the selection of foods, cooking methods, cooking times, the water content of the various dishes, and the cutting methods and seasonings used, the cook can continually build health and vitality, while adapting to the changing environment.

The cook's attitude also affects the quality of the meal he or she is preparing. A calm, peaceful mind is important while preparing and serving food. All distractions, problems, and stresses are best put aside when you enter the kitchen.

To cook in a natural, balanced way, it is important to be sensitive to the surrounding environment. Being aware of the changing seasons and learning how to adapt to them is a necessary part of this. For example, during the spring and summer it is better to use shorter cooking times and to serve light, fresh dishes. These help balance our condition with hotter weather. As we approach autumn and winter, it is appropriate for our cooking to change to include more warming factors, such as a little more salt, oil, and other seasonings, and a greater number of hearty, well-cooked dishes like thick soups and stews. Daily weather conditions are also important. For example, on wet, rainy days, less water is needed in cooking; more can be added on dry, hot days.

The quality of fire used in cooking also plays a vital role in health and well-being. For most people, gas ranges are the most practical and healthful fuel source. They provide a clean, even, easily controllable flame. Many people who have changed to a natural diet have also converted from electric to gas cooking. Most report improvements in their cooking and the flavor of their foods, as well as in their energy levels and overall health.

For those with electric stoves who are unable to install a gas range right away, small portable propane gas stoves can be used in the kitchen along with an electric range. These portable units have several burners, and can be used in preparing pressure-cooked rice, miso soup, and other staples, while side dishes can be prepared on the electric range. Microwave ovens are not recommended for healthful cooking.

WASHING FOOD

It is better not to wash and cut foods too long before you are ready to use them, as this causes them to lose freshness and nutritional value. Wash vegetables before cutting them, because vegetables that are cut before being washed lose taste and nutrients.

Foods such as whole grains, beans, seeds, vegetables, sea-vegetables, and fruits can be quickly washed with cold water. This causes the skin, shell, or outer portion of the food to contract and helps prevent nutrient loss. Foods washed with warm water are often bland-tasting. More specific guidelines for washing various types of food are provided below.

Washing Grains, Beans, and Seeds. Before washing these foods, first sort them to remove any small stones, clumps of soil, or badly damaged pieces. Place the grains, beans, or seeds in a bowl, place the bowl in the sink, and fill it with water beyond the level of the food. Rinse by stirring gently with your fingers, and pour the water off. Repeat the process again, and then transfer the food, a handful at a time, to a strainer. Rinse quickly under cold water. Your grains, beans, or seeds are now ready to be cooked or roasted.

Washing Vegetables and Fruits. Leafy green vegetables, especially those with jagged edges like kale and carrot greens, can be held under cold running water or soaked in a bowl of cold water for several seconds. An entire bunch of greens can be rinsed or soaked in this way. Then, wash each leaf by hand under cold running water. Most leafy greens require thorough washing before they are ready to cook. Larger leaves, like cabbage or Chinese cabbage, can be washed individually after you separate them from the core.

Root and round vegetables can be cleaned with a natural bristle vegetable brush, as can fruits. Scrub firmly but gently to remove soil. Be careful not to remove the skin while scrubbing. The skin of vegetables and fruits is best kept on, as it contains nutrients that are a part of the whole food. Onions are an exception; they can be peeled and quickly rinsed under cold water before slicing. Of course, produce that has been waxed or overly chemicalized requires peeling or at least thorough scrubbing.

Washing Sea-Vegetables. Plants from the sea sometimes have tiny stones or shells attached to them; these are easy to remove by hand. Most sea-vegetables can be washed in the manner described for grains and seeds. After washing, they are generally best soaked for about five minutes (until they become soft enough to slice smoothly). An exception to this is arame. This sea-vegetable is shredded before being dried, and it loses sweetness and flavor when it is soaked. It is better to simply wash arame and allow it to absorb the water that remains from washing. Also, kombu is normally wiped with a clean damp towel or sponge instead of being washed before soaking. Three to five minutes is normally all that is required when soaking sea-vegetables.

THE ART OF CUTTING

We recommend using a variety of cutting methods whenever you cook in order to create attractive and delicious dishes. As you familiarize yourself with the recipes in this book, you will discover that some dishes, like nishime, require thicker, more chunky cuts, while others, like kinpira, require fine and delicate cuts. With practice, anyone can learn to cut vegetables in an artistic and balanced fashion.

When cutting vegetables, do not cut straight down or use your knife like a saw. Start with the front tip or edge, and gently slide the length of the blade across the vegetable in one smooth stroke. Keep your fingertips curled so that your knuckles rest against the knife. This protects against accidental cuts and slips and helps you get a better grip on the vegetable.

The cutting methods used in this book, including diagonal slices, half-moons, matchsticks, and triangular shapes, are illustrated in Figure 3.1, following.

OTHER BASICS

Along with the methods of cutting, washing, and prepping foods presented above, some additional basics are helpful when beginning to cook macrobiotically. These include:

How to Soak Dried Foods

Many of the foods recommended in macrobiotic cooking are bought dried, and require soaking before being cooked. Some of the dried foods that are often soaked include:

Sea-Vegetables (including kombu, wakame, hiziki, dulse, and sea palm): After washing, place the sea-vegetable in a bowl and add enough cold water to just cover it. Let the sea-vegetable soak for 3–5 minutes, remove, drain, and slice. If the soaking water is very salty, discard it. Otherwise, use it in cooking as part of your water measurement.

Dried Daikon: Rinse the dried, shredded daikon quickly under cold water. Place it in a bowl and add just enough cold water to cover. Let it soak for 5–10 minutes. Remove, squeeze out excess liquid, and slice. If the soaking water is very dark, discard it. If it is lighter in color, you may use it as part of your water measurement in cooking.

Figure 3.1   Cutting Methods

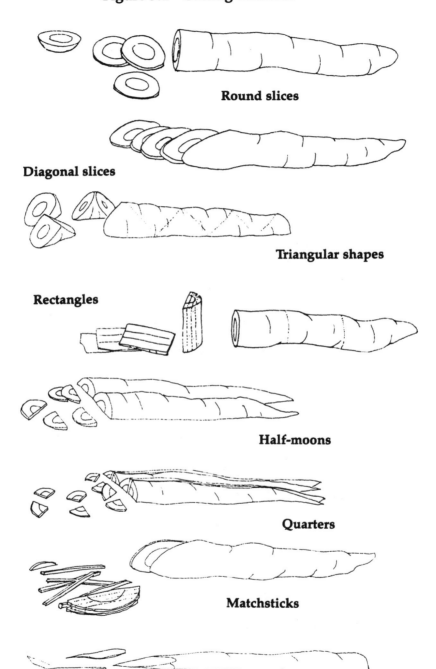

Round slices

Diagonal slices

Triangular shapes

Rectangles

Half-moons

Quarters

Matchsticks

Shavings

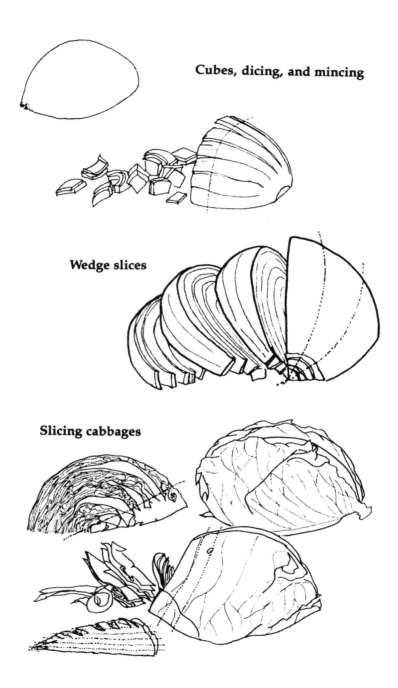

Cubes, dicing, and mincing

Wedge slices

Slicing cabbages

Slicing big, leafy greens

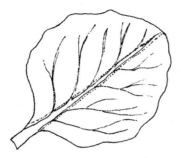

Along the veins

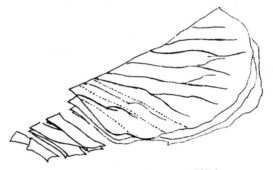

Slicing greens

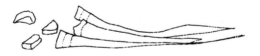

The stem

Dried Tofu: Place dried tofu in a bowl and add warm water to cover. Let it soak for 7–10 minutes. Remove, rinse under cold water, and squeeze out liquid. Slice as indicated in the recipe. The soaking water from dried tofu can be discarded.

Shiitake Mushrooms: Place the shiitake in a bowl and add warm water to cover. Let them soak for 10–15 minutes. Remove, squeeze out liquid, and remove the stems. Slice the shiitake as instructed in the recipe. The stems may be used in preparing soup stock and then discarded. The soaking water may be used as part of your water measurement in cooking.

Dried Lotus Seeds: Rinse the seeds quickly under cold water. Place them in a bowl and add cold water to cover. Let them soak for ½–1 hour. Remove and use as instructed in the recipe. The soaking water may be used as a part of your water measurement.

Dried Fu: Place the fu in a bowl and add enough cold water to cover. Let it soak for 5–10 minutes. Remove, squeeze out the liquid, and slice as indicated in the recipe. The soaking water may be used in cooking.

Dried Chestnuts: Rinse the chestnuts quickly under cold water. Then, dry roast them in a dry skillet until golden brown. Place in a bowl and add enough cold water to just cover. Let them soak for 10–15 minutes. Remove and use as indicated in the recipe. The soaking water may be used as part of the water measurement in the recipe.

Dried Fruit: Rinse dried fruit quickly under cold water. Place in a bowl and add just enough cold water to cover. Soak for 10–15 minutes until soft. Remove and squeeze out liquid. Slice or cook whole as per recipe instructions. The soaking water may be used in cooking.

Whole Grains: After washing your grains in cold water, place them in a bowl or pressure cooker. Add the required amount of water—as instructed in the recipe—and soak, without salt, for 6–8 hours. Whole grains can be cooked in their soaking water.

Beans: Wash beans in cold water. Place them in a bowl and add enough cold water to cover. Let them soak for 6–8 hours. Remove and drain. If you are cooking low-fat beans such as azuki, chickpeas, or black soybeans, you may use the soaking water as a part of the recipe. The soaking water from other beans may be discarded.

How to Dilute Powdered Foods

Several of the foods used in macrobiotic cooking come in a powdered form. They need to be diluted with water before being used in recipes.

Kuzu: Place kuzu in a cup and add an equal amount of cold water. Stir until completely dissolved.

Arrowroot Flour: Place arrowroot flour in a cup and add slightly more water than flour. Stir until completely dissolved.

Puréeing Miso for Soups

Miso, a frequent ingredient used in seasoning soup, is puréed before being added to the stock. This helps it to dissolve more thoroughly and allows it to mix more completely in the broth. To purée miso, place it in a suribachi and add the same—or a slightly larger—amount of water or broth from the soup. Purée until it is thoroughly dissolved and has a smooth consistency.

Grating Ginger or Daikon

Grated ginger or grated daikon are used in cooking as well as in preparing special drinks and home care. To grate properly, use a flat stainless steel or porcelain grater and grate the amount called for in the recipe. If you are going to use the juice and not the pulp, simply place the gratings in your hand and squeeze the juice into a bowl. Discard the pulp or save for use in another recipe.

Unfamiliar Cooking Methods

Some of the cooking methods—such as pressure cooking, steaming, boiling, and sautéing—are generally well known and are used often by cooks today. However, some of the methods introduced in this book may be new and unfamiliar. Below is a short explanation of these methods for those who are unfamiliar with macrobiotic cooking.

Water Sautéing: To water sauté, place enough water in a skillet to just cover the bottom. Heat up. Add vegetables and sauté as you would with oil. If the water evaporates, simply add a small amount as needed until the vegetables are finished cooking.

Nishime: This is a method of slow boiling in which vegetables are cut into large pieces. It uses a very small amount of water, and the vegetables are cooked over a low flame for about 40–45 minutes. This method is often referred to as "waterless cooking" since vegetables are cooked until the liquid evaporates. The vegetables are not stirred or mixed until they are nearly finished cooking.

Kinpira: This cooking method uses elements of boiling and sautéing. The vegetables are first sautéed and then boiled or simmered. Any liquid that remains is cooked away near the end.

Ohitashi: Ohitashi is another method of boiling that is used mostly for leafy green vegetables. The vegetables may be sliced or left whole. Water is brought to a boil, and the vegetables are added and boiled from several seconds to a minute. This method is sometimes referred to as "blanching."

SAVING TIME AND ENERGY

Once you begin cooking, you will discover many shortcuts to help save time and energy in the kitchen. One way to save time is to plan ahead so that all of the dishes in a meal will be finished cooking at the same time. Start the dishes that require the longest time first, and those with shorter cooking times later. If, for example, your meal includes brown rice, soup, steamed greens, beans, a sea-vegetable dish, and a pickle or pressed salad, start the beans first, as they need the longest time to cook. Then put up your pressed salad, as it needs to sit for an hour or so before it is ready. Meanwhile, start your rice, and then move on to the sea-vegetable or soup. Steamed greens take only a few minutes to cook, so they can be started last.

Once your dishes are cooking, you can save energy by letting the foods cook themselves! Don't look into the cooking pots too often or stir your foods unnecessarily. Simply check them now and then to make sure they are coming along properly.

PLANNING MENUS

Preparing a complete meal may require advance planning, especially while the foods and cooking methods are still unfamiliar to you. It is a challenge to select and cook dishes that complement each other as a part of a balanced meal. With time, however, your ability to do this will become intuitive and natural.

In the next chapter, we present complete breakfast, lunch, and dinner menus for a seven-day period. The recipes have been carefully selected and arranged to balance taste, energy, and daily requirements within the standard macrobiotic diet. These basic menus can serve as an introduction to the preparation of balanced natural meals. As you become comfortable in the kitchen, feel free to expand your horizons and create new and exciting meals using the full range of whole natural foods.

Chapter Four

A SEVEN-DAY MENU PLAN

In this chapter we present menus and recipes for one week of complete natural food meals. The menus are arranged so that you can have maximum flexibility in meal selection, and designed to help you become comfortable with macrobiotic cooking.

The seven breakfast menus are presented in a group, as are the lunches and dinners. Each menu is followed by recipes that feature clear, step-by-step instructions for preparing each item.

The Seven-Day Menu Plan can be used any number of ways. One way is to try all of the menus as they appear in the book—for example, starting with Menu 1 for breakfast, Menu 1 for lunch, and Menu 1 for dinner, and continuing with Menu 2, Menu 3, and so forth. Alternatively, you can vary the order and combine the menus according to your preference, for example, Breakfast Menu 3, Lunch Menu 5, and Dinner Menu 1. Over 300 menu combinations are possible with this approach.

Another way you can use this menu plan is to try individual menus or dishes. This approach can be equally useful for those making a gradual transition to natural foods and for those who are already cooking this way. Regardless of your cooking experience, preparing the dishes in this chapter will help you discover the art of preparing balanced natural meals.

Feel free to be creative in designing your menus and cooking. As you develop healthful new dishes, add them to the menus to create your own meal plan. Ingredients in the recipes can also be changed, depending on your tastes and preferences. In many instances, we have included suggestions for varying the recipes. Keep in mind that flexibility, change, and variety are the keys to successful macrobiotic cooking and are basic to good health.

BALANCED BREAKFASTS

In the daily cycle, morning is the time of rising energy. Foods with a similar quality—light and simple—are best at this time. Whole grain porridges, made by cooking grains with more water than usual (so that they become soft and creamy) are very good as the center of the morning meal. Mildly seasoned miso soup, simply made, is also very good at breakfast. The kind of miso used most often in macrobiotic cooking is made from barley (a grain known for its rising energy) fermented with soybeans and sea salt. Fermentation gives miso a more expansive quality.

Quickly cooked or pickled vegetables can also be served at breakfast, and they often are in traditional diets. In general, a large, heavy breakfast—with many fatty foods and plenty of sugar—promotes disharmony with the natural energy of the environment.

The seven menus offer suggestions for satisfying breakfasts that are quick and simple to prepare. We hope you will enjoy them.

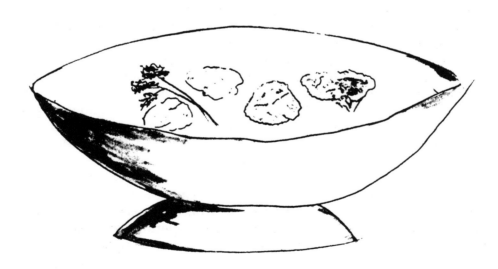

Breakfast

Menu One

Miso Soup with Onions and Wakame

Soft Rice with Umeboshi

Toasted Nori Squares

Steamed Kale

Bancha Tea

Miso Soup with Onions and Wakame

4–5 cups water
1/2 cup wakame, washed, soaked,
   and sliced
2 cups onions, sliced in
   half-moons
1/4–1/2 teaspoon puréed barley
   miso per cup of liquid

Yield: Four to five servings.

Place the water in a pot and bring it to a boil. Add the wakame and simmer for 1–2 minutes. Add the onions and cover the pot. Simmer until tender, approximately 2–3 minutes. Reduce the flame to low and simmer until the onions are soft and translucent. Then reduce the flame to very low so that there is no bubbling action. Add enough puréed miso to the soup pot to create a mild salt taste. Simmer over a very low flame, with a flame deflector under the pot, for another 3–4 minutes. Place the soup in individual serving bowls and garnish with a few sliced scallions or chopped parsley. Serve hot.

Soft Rice with Umeboshi

1 cup organic brown rice
5 cups water
1 umeboshi plum
sliced scallions

Yield: Four to five servings.

Wash the rice and place it in the pressure cooker. Add the water and the umeboshi plum. Cover the cooker, turn the flame to high, and bring up the cooker to pressure. Place a flame deflector under the cooker when the pressure is up. Reduce the flame to low and pressure cook for approximately 50–60 minutes. Remove from the flame and allow pressure to come down slowly. Remove the cover when all pressure is out of the cooker. Place the rice in individual serving bowls; garnish with sliced scallions or your favorite condiment, and serve hot.

Toasted Nori Squares

2 sheets nori sea-vegetable

Yield: Four to five servings.

Toasted nori goes well with many dishes and is often used as a garnish. To toast nori for general use, turn the flame to high. Take 1 sheet and hold it 10–12 inches above the flame so that the inside fold of the sheet faces downward. Rotate the sheet over the flame so that it toasts evenly. In a few seconds, it will change from dark green or black to a bright green color. Cut the sheet into quarters, stacking them on top of each other. Then, with a pair of scissors, cut the toasted nori into squares or strips. Use it as a garnish for soft rice, soups, stews, or noodle dishes; or wrap it around toasted mochi (see page 62).

Steamed Kale

2–3 cups kale, washed and sliced
water

Yield: Four to five servings.

Place about ½ inch of water in a pot. Set a steamer basket down inside the pot or place a bamboo steamer on top. Bring the water to a boil. Place the kale in the steamer, cover, and steam until the kale is tender but still slightly crisp and has a bright green color. Remove, drain, and place in a serving dish.

Instead of slicing the kale first, you can steam or boil 4–5 whole leaves and then slice them when they're done. This way of cooking vegetables—especially greens—is delicious because it keeps most of the natural juices and nutrients from getting lost during cooking.

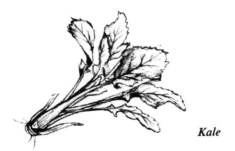

Kale

Bancha Tea

1 tablespoon bancha twigs
1 quart water

Yield: Four to five servings.

For a strong beverage, first place the twigs in a dry stainless steel skillet and roast them for several minutes. For a lighter tea, simply place the twigs in a teakettle without roasting. Add the water and place the kettle over a high flame. Bring to a boil, then reduce the flame to low. For a mild tea, simmer 2–3 minutes. You can simmer the twigs for up to 10 minutes if you prefer strong tea. Serve hot.

Menu Two

Soft Millet with Squash and Cabbage

Broiled Tofu

Gomashio

Boiled Mustard Greens

Grain Coffee

Soft Millet with Squash and Cabbage

1 cup millet
4 cups water
1 cup buttercup or butternut
   squash or Hokkaido pumpkin,
   cut into 1–2 inch cubes (leave
   skin on if organic or unwaxed)
1 cup green cabbage, washed
   and cut into 1–2 inch chunks
pinch of sea salt

Yield: Four to five servings.

Wash and drain the millet. Place it in a dry, heated skillet. Dry roast over a low flame for several minutes, until the millet is golden brown and releases a nutty fragrance. Stir constantly to prevent burning. Remove the millet and place in a pressure cooker. Add water, squash, cabbage, and sea salt. Cover the cooker and place it over a high flame. Bring up to pressure. When the pressure is up, reduce the flame to medium-low and place a flame deflector under the cooker. Cook for approximately 15–20 minutes. Remove from the flame and allow the pressure to come down. Remove the cover, place the millet in individual serving bowls, and garnish each bowl with a small amount of freshly-made gomashio (see below) and a few sliced scallions. Serve hot.

Broiled Tofu

8–10 slices fresh tofu, each about
  ¹/₂ inch thick by 2 inches wide
  by 3 inches long
tamari soy sauce

Yield: Four to five servings.

Place the sliced tofu on a dry baking- or cookie sheet. Sprinkle a little tamari soy sauce on top of each slice. Turn on the broiler and place the tofu under it. Broil for 4–5 minutes or until the tofu is slightly browned but moist. Turn the slices over and again sprinkle with a small amount of tamari soy sauce. Place the tofu back under the broiler and broil for another 4–5 minutes or until slightly brown but moist. Place the broiled tofu on a serving dish, garnish with a sprig of parsley or a little sauerkraut, and serve.

Gomashio

16 tablespoons sesame seeds (tan
  or black), washed and drained
1 tablespoon sea salt

Yield: Four to five servings.

While the sesame seeds are still damp, place them in a dry, heated stainless steel skillet. Roast over a medium-low flame. Stir constantly with a wooden spoon or bamboo rice paddle to evenly roast and prevent burning. Occasionally shake the skillet back and forth to further ensure even roasting. The seeds are ready when they give off a nutty fragrance, turn golden brown in color, and begin to pop slightly. When the seeds are done they can easily be crushed between your thumb and little finger. Pour the roasted seeds into a bowl. Place the sea salt in a heated dry skillet and roast it for 2–3 minutes. Transfer the roasted sea salt to a suribachi and grind to a smooth, fine powder. Add the roasted sesame seeds and slowly grind with an even circular motion, using the sides of the suribachi, until each sesame seed is about half-crushed. Allow the gomashio to cool before placing it in a container that can be tightly sealed for storage. Sprinkle gomashio lightly over grains, or on vegetable or noodle dishes as a condiment.

Boiled Mustard Greens

1 small bunch mustard greens,
   washed and left whole
water

Yield: Four to five servings.

Place about ½ inch of water in a pot and bring it to a boil. Place the whole mustard greens in the pot; cover and boil for 1–2 minutes, until they're tender but still bright green in color. Remove the greens, place them in a colander or strainer, and allow them to drain and cool. If you want to retain a very dark or bright green color, you may run the greens under cold water for several seconds. However, for optimum flavor it is better to spread the greens out and let them cool naturally. Slice the greens into 1-inch pieces and place them in a serving bowl.

Grain Coffee

1 teaspoon grain coffee
1 cup boiling water

Yield: Four to five servings.

Instant grain coffee can be found in most natural food stores, but if you can't locate it, you can prepare your own by individually roasting barley, rice, azuki beans, chickpeas, burdock, or chicory, etc., and grinding them (again, individually) to a very fine powder in a grain mill. Combine the various ingredients once they have been ground. To prepare instant grain coffee, put a teaspoonful in a cup and pour boiling water over it. Stir and drink. Homemade grain coffee can be brewed in a coffeepot or simmered for several minutes in a saucepan.

=====================================

Menu Three

=====================================

Miso Soft Rice

Boiled Chinese Cabbage Rolls with Umeboshi Paste

Pickled Turnips and Kombu

Brown Rice Tea

=====================================

Miso Soft Rice

1 strip kombu, 4–5 inches long,
  soaked and diced
2 shiitake mushrooms, soaked,
  de-stemmed, and diced
1 teaspoon finely minced scallion
  roots
1 cup daikon, washed,
  quartered, and thinly sliced
1 cup organic brown rice,
  washed
5 cups water
1/2 cup chopped scallions
1/2–1 teaspoon puréed barley
  miso per cup of cooked grain

Yield: Four to five servings.

Place the kombu, shiitake, scallion roots, daikon, rice, and water in a pressure cooker. Put the cover on the cooker, turn the flame to high and bring the cooker up to pressure. Reduce the flame to medium-low and simmer for approximately 50–60 minutes. Remove the pressure cooker from the flame and allow the pressure to come down. Remove the cover and place the cooker over a low flame. Add the appropriate amount of miso for a mild salt taste, and add the chopped scallions. Mix the miso and scallions in with the rice and simmer over a very low flame for 3–4 minutes. Place each portion in an individual serving bowl and garnish with a small amount of chopped scallion or parsley. Serve hot.

Boiled Chinese Cabbage Rolls with Umeboshi Paste

9–12 medium-large Chinese
  cabbage leaves
1 carrot, 8–10 inches long,
  quartered lengthwise
1 teaspoon umeboshi paste
water

Yield: Four to five servings.

Place about 1 inch of water in a pot and bring it to a boil. Place the Chinese cabbage leaves in the pot and cover. Boil the Chinese cabbage 2–3 minutes, until it is basically tender but still firm and slightly crisp. Carefully remove the Chinese cabbage and spread it out in a colander to drain and cool. Place the carrot strips in the same boiling water, cover, and simmer for 1–2 minutes, or until tender. Remove the carrot strips and let them drain and cool.

To assemble the sushi, refer to Figure 4.1, following. Place a bamboo sushi mat on a cutting board. Place 2 cabbage leaves across the mat in alternate directions, with the hard stem parts facing out toward the sides of the mat. Then take 2 more leaves and place them on top of the first leaves so that they cover about half of the bottom layer of the original leaves. Place 1 strip of carrot in the center of leaves, so that it spans the entire length of the leaves.

Pull up the sushi mat slightly with your fingers and press firmly against the cabbage leaves. Hold the mat with your thumbs and index fingers. With your other fingers, tuck the cabbage leaves under as you roll them up. Continue to roll up the sushi mat, pressing firmly to produce a tightly rolled cylinder of leaves. When the leaves are completely rolled into a cylinder, wrap the sushi mat around them tightly and firmly squeeze the roll to remove any excess liquid.

Remove the sushi mat and place the cabbage roll on a cutting board. With a sharp knife, slice the cabbage roll in half. Then slice each half into 4 equal-sized pieces about 1 inch long. Stand each slice on end on a serving platter so that the carrot is displayed in the center. Place a small dab of umeboshi paste on top of each piece. Repeat with the remaining cabbage leaves and carrots. For variety, other large leafy greens, such as kale, collards, chard, or mustard greens can be rolled in the same way.

Figure 4.1 Boiled Chinese Cabbage Rolls With Umeboshi Paste

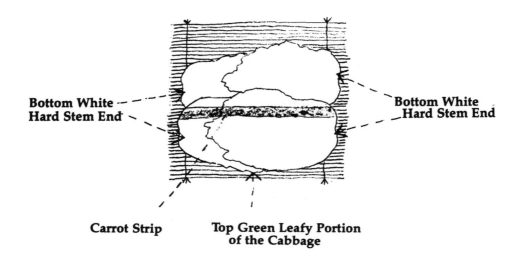

Bottom White --
Hard Stem End ~

Bottom White
_Hard Stem End

Carrot Strip   Top Green Leafy Portion
                         of the Cabbage

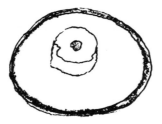

Rolled Up View (Then slice where indicated.)

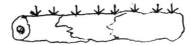

Cross Section View After Sliced and Stood on End

Pickled Turnips and Kombu

1 medium turnip, washed,
    quartered, and very thinly
    sliced (1½–2 cups sliced)
1 strip kombu, soaked and sliced
    into very thin matchsticks
1 teaspoon sea salt

Yield: Four to five servings.

Place the kombu, turnips, and sea salt in a pickle press and mix them very well. Place the top on the press and screw it down firmly to apply pressure. When water is expelled from the pickles and rises above the pressure plate, release the pressure slightly until the water level drops just below the plate. Let the pickles sit for 1–2 days. If the pickled turnips are too salty, rinse them quickly under cold water before serving. They will keep about 1 week if stored in a cool place or in the refrigerator.

Brown Rice Tea

½ cup brown rice, washed
1 quart water

Yield: Four to five servings.

Heat up a dry skillet. Place the rice in the skillet and roast it until it turns golden brown, stirring constantly to evenly roast and prevent burning. Remove the rice and place it in a teakettle with 1 quart of water. Bring the water to a boil, reduce the flame to low, and simmer for approximately 15–20 minutes. Strain through a tea strainer and serve hot.

As a variation, try other grains such as barley or hato mugi (unroasted pearl barley), or combine roasted rice with a small amount of bancha twigs (see recipe on page 67). Tea made from brown rice and barley (see page 63) is also very refreshing any time of day.

Menu Four

Daikon-Shiitake Miso Soup

Toasted Mochi Wrapped in Nori

Grated Daikon

Boiled Tempeh with Leeks

Barley Tea

Daikon-Shiitake Miso Soup

4–5 cups water
3 shiitake mushrooms, soaked,
   de-stemmed, and sliced
1/4 cup wakame, washed, soaked
   2–3 minutes, and sliced
1 cup daikon, washed and sliced
   in thin half-moons
1/2–1 teaspoon puréed barley
   miso per cup of liquid
sliced scallions or parsley

Yield: Four to five servings.

Place the water in a pot and bring it to a boil. Add the shiitake mushrooms, cover, and simmer for 10–15 minutes. Add the wakame, cover, and simmer 2–3 minutes. Next place the daikon in the water, cover, and simmer 2–3 minutes (until tender). Reduce the flame to very low and add the puréed miso. Simmer for 2–3 minutes longer. Place the soup in individual serving bowls. Garnish and serve hot. As a variation, place a piece of toasted mochi (see below) in the hot soup.

Toasted Mochi Wrapped in Nori

6–8 slices of mochi, approxi-
    mately 3 inches by 2 inches
1 sheet toasted nori, cut into
    strips 4 inches long by 1–1½
    inches wide
tamari soy sauce

Yield: Four to five servings.

Place the sliced mochi in a dry skillet over a low flame. Cover the skillet
and toast the mochi until it turns golden brown. Be careful not to let it
burn. Turn the mochi over and brown the other side. It may take 3–5
minutes to toast the mochi on each side. Wrap a strip of nori around
each piece of mochi, sealing the ends together with a drop of water.
Serve several pieces of mochi to each person. When eating, you may
place 1–2 drops of tamari soy sauce on each piece. You may also place a
dab of grated daikon (see below) on the mochi to aid in digestion.

Instead of roasting mochi in a skillet, try baking it for several minutes
until it puffs up, or even broiling it for 3–4 minutes. If you're broiling
the mochi, be careful that it does not burn. Toasted mochi is a good addition to miso soup. This makes a very delicious and strengthening
soup, especially in colder weather.

Grated Daikon

1 piece daikon root, 4–6 inches
    long, washed
tamari soy sauce

Yield: Four to five servings.

Grate the daikon on a flat grater and place it in a small dish (there will
be about ½ cup). Garnish with several drops of tamari soy sauce and a
few scallion slices. Eat grated daikon with mochi (or with seafood or
fried dishes) to aid digestion.

Boiled Tempeh with Leeks

2 cups tempeh, sliced into 1-inch
    cubes
1–1½ cups leeks, washed and
    sliced on a diagonal into pieces
    about ¼ inch thick
tamari soy sauce
water

Yield: Four to five servings.

Place the tempeh in a skillet and add enough water to about half cover.
Cover the skillet and bring to a boil. Reduce the flame to medium-low
and simmer about 20–25 minutes. Add the leeks and a small amount of
tamari soy sauce. Cover and simmer until the leeks are tender but still
bright green. Remove the cover and cook off the remaining liquid. Mix
and place in a serving bowl.

You can also try making boiled tempeh with sliced scallions instead of
leeks, with sauerkraut and sliced cabbage, or with any other vegetables
you wish. Season with umeboshi or a little umeboshi vinegar for a
different flavor.

Barley Tea

1 tablespoon roasted barley
1 quart water

Yield: Four to five servings.

Prepackaged, roasted, unhulled barley for making tea can be purchased
in most natural food stores. It is sold under the name mugi-cha. You can
also make homemade barley tea by roasting barley in a dry skillet over a
low flame until it turns golden brown. Stir constantly to evenly roast
the barley and prevent burning.

Place the roasted barley in a kettle filled with 1 quart of water. Bring
the water to a boil, reduce the flame to low, and simmer to desired
strength. For a mild tea try simmering for 3–5 minutes; for a stronger
flavor, simmer 10–15 minutes. In the summer months this tea is very
refreshing when slightly chilled and served with a slice of lemon on the
side.

Menu Five

Whole Oats

Toasted Rice Bread

Onion Butter

Sautéed Celery and Carrots

Goma-Dulse Powder

Bancha Tea

Whole Oats

1 cup whole oats, washed
4 cups water
pinch of sea salt

Yield: Four to five servings.

Place the whole oats, water, and sea salt in a pressure cooker and cover. Place over a high flame and bring up to pressure. Reduce the flame to medium-low and simmer for about 1 hour. Remove the cooker from the flame and allow the pressure to come down. When all the pressure is out, remove the cover and place the oats in individual serving bowls. Garnish with goma-dulse powder (see below) a few raisins, a natural sweetener, or any favorite condiment.

Whole oats may be prepared in a variety of ways. They can be soaked overnight before cooking, or even dry-roasted, for a different favor. Whole oats may be boiled instead of pressure cooked, if desired. This may take 2–3 hours. Sometimes sliced onions are very nice when cooked with the oats. Dried fruit can occasionally be cooked with oats for a sweet flavor.

Toasted Rice Bread

> 6–8 slices rice bread (or other
>   whole grain bread)

Yield: Six to eight servings.

Simply toast the bread and serve it with onion butter (see below) or another favorite spread.

Onion Butter

> 10 medium onions, diced or
>   finely minced
> dark sesame oil (optional)
> pinch of sea salt
> water

Yield: Four to five servings.

Heat a small amount of dark sesame oil in a large pot or deep skillet. (You may water-sauté the onions if you wish to avoid oil.) Add the onions and sauté them over a medium-low flame until they become translucent. Stir occasionally to prevent burning and to evenly sauté. Add a pinch of sea salt and enough water to just cover the onions. Cover and bring to a boil. Reduce the flame to very low and simmer for several hours, until the onions become dark brown in color, are very sweet, and have almost melted. There should not be any liquid left when the onion butter is done. You may occasionally add a small amount of water to prevent burning. You may spread warm onion butter on whole grain bread or toast, or allow it to cool and keep some on hand. Store it in a glass jar that is tightly sealed and kept in a cool place or refrigerator.

Try onion butter on rice cakes or crackers for a treat. Carrots and squash can be cooked in the same manner. For variety, you may also combine onions with these vegetables.

Sautéed Celery and Carrots

1 cup celery, thinly sliced on a
   diagonal
2 cups carrots, sliced into thin
   matchsticks
dark sesame oil
pinch of sea salt or several drops
   of tamari soy sauce
water

Yield: Four to five servings.

Heat a small amount of dark sesame oil in a skillet. Place the celery in
the skillet and sauté 1–2 minutes. Then add the carrots and sauté another 1–2 minutes. Add a pinch of sea salt or several drops of tamari
soy sauce and enough water to just cover the bottom of the skillet.
Cover and bring to a boil. Reduce the flame to low and simmer until the
vegetables are tender. Remove the cover and cook off any remaining
liquid. Place in a serving dish.

Goma-Dulse Powder

1/2 cup dried dulse (Do not
   wash.)
1/2 cup tan sesame seeds, washed
   and roasted

Yield: Four to five servings.

Place the dulse on a cookie sheet and bake in the oven for 15–20 minutes at 350°F, until crisp but not burnt. Remove the dulse and place it in
a suribachi. Grind it to a fine powder. Add the roasted sesame seeds
and grind them together with the dulse powder until each seed is about
half-crushed. Serve goma-dulse powder on hot cereal as a condiment.
To store, allow the goma-dulse powder to cool and place it in a glass or
ceramic container that can be tightly sealed.

Bancha Tea

> 1 tablespoon bancha twigs
> 1 quart water
>
> Yield: Four to five servings.

For a strong beverage, first place the twigs in a dry stainless steel skillet and roast them for several minutes. For a lighter tea, simply place the twigs in a teakettle without roasting. Add the water and place the kettle over a high flame. Bring to a boil, then reduce the flame to low. For a mild tea, simmer 2–3 minutes. You can simmer the twigs for up to 10 minutes if you prefer strong tea. Serve hot.

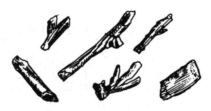

Bancha tea

Menu Six

Soft Barley and Shiitake

Shiso-Green Nori Flake Condiment

Sautéed Chinese Cabbage and Kale

Grain Coffee

Soft Barley and Shiitake

5–6 shiitake mushrooms, soaked,
  de-stemmed, and diced
water from soaking shiitake
1 cup onions, diced
1/2 cup celery, diced
1/4 cup dried daikon, soaked and
  sliced
1 strip kombu, 3–4 inches long,
  soaked and diced
1 cup barley, soaked 6–8 hours
5 cups water
pinch of sea salt
sliced scallions
tamari soy sauce (optional)

Yield: Four to five servings.

Place the shiitake, the water from soaking the shiitake, the shiitake, the
onions, the celery, the dried daikon, and the kombu in a pressure
cooker. Add the soaked barley, water, and a pinch of sea salt. Cover and
place over a high flame. When the pressure is up, reduce the flame to
medium-low and cook for approximately 50 minutes. Remove the
cooker from the flame and allow the pressure to come down. Remove
the cover and spoon the barley mixture into individual serving bowls.
Garnish with a few sliced scallions and a drop or two of tamari soy
sauce, if desired.

Shiso-Green Nori Flake Condiment

1/4 cup shiso leaves
1/2 cup green nori flakes (Ao nori)
1/2 cup tan sesame seeds, roasted

Yield: Four to five servings.

Chop the shiso leaves very fine and dry-roast them in a skillet for several minutes, until dry. Place the shiso in a suribachi and grind to a fine
powder. Add the roasted sesame seeds and grind until half-crushed.
Mix in the green nori flakes. Serve this condiment over grains or soft

cereals. To store, allow it to cool and seal it tightly in a glass or ceramic container.

Sautéed Chinese Cabbage and Kale

3 cups Chinese cabbage, washed
   and thickly sliced on a diagonal
1 cup kale, washed and sliced on
   a diagonal
dark sesame oil
pinch of sea salt or several drops
   of tamari soy sauce

Yield: Four to five servings.

Place a small amount of dark sesame oil in a skillet and heat. Add the Chinese cabbage and kale. Add a small pinch of sea salt. Sauté for 1–2 minutes. Add a few drops of tamari soy sauce, cover, and sauté several minutes more, until the vegetables become tender but are still bright green in color. You will need to stir occasionally. Remove and place in a serving dish.

Grain Coffee

1 teaspoon grain coffee
1 cup boiling water

Yield: One serving.

Instant grain coffee can be found in most natural food stores, but if you can't locate it, you can prepare your own by individually roasting barley, rice, azuki beans, chickpeas, burdock, or chicory, etc., and grinding them (again, individually) to a very fine powder in a grain mill. Combine the various ingredients once they have been ground. To prepare instant grain coffee, put a teaspoonful in a cup and pour boiling water over it. Stir and drink. Homemade grain coffee can be brewed in a coffeepot or simmered for several minutes in a saucepan.

Menu Seven

Daikon-Celery Miso Soup

Tofu French Toast

Lemon-Rice Syrup Topping

Apple-Raisin Kuzu Topping

Mochi Waffles

Steamed Collard Greens

Barley Tea

Daikon-Celery Miso Soup

4–5 cups water
1/4 cup wakame, soaked and
   sliced
2 cups daikon, quartered and
   thinly sliced
1 cup celery, thickly sliced on a
   diagonal
1/2–1 teaspoon puréed barley
   miso per cup of liquid
chopped parsley

Yield: Four to five servings.

Place the water in a pot and bring to a boil. Add the wakame and boil
1–2 minutes. Add the celery and boil 1–2 minutes. Then place the
daikon in the water, cover, and reduce the flame to medium-low. Simmer until the vegetables are tender. Reduce the flame to very low and

add the puréed miso. Cover and simmer 2–3 minutes. Place the soup in individual serving bowls and garnish with chopped parsley.

Tofu French Toast

1 cake tofu (1 pound)
1/2 cup water
1 teaspoon tamari soy sauce
8 slices whole wheat bread
dark sesame or corn oil

Yield: Four to five servings.

Place the tofu, water, and tamari soy sauce in a blender and blend to a creamy consistency. Heat a small amount of dark sesame oil in a skillet. Pour the creamed tofu into a large bowl. Dip the slices of bread into the tofu mixture, covering both sides lightly. Fry the tofu-coated bread until golden brown. Flip the toast over and fry the other side until golden brown; then remove it and place it on a serving platter. Repeat until all the ingredients are used up. Serve with one of the recipes listed below or another favorite topping.

Lemon-Rice Syrup Topping

1/2 cup rice syrup
2 tablespoons water
1/2 teaspoon fresh-squeezed
lemon juice

Yield: Four to five servings.

Place all the ingredients in a saucepan and heat up. Then place the topping in a serving container and pour it over Tofu French toast or Mochi Waffles (see below).

Apple-Raisin Kuzu Topping

¼ cup raisins, soaked 15 minutes
    or so
2 apples, washed and sliced
2 cups apple juice (or 1 cup water
    and 1 cup juice)
pinch of sea salt
2 heaping teaspoons kuzu

Yield: Four to five servings.

Place the raisins, apples, apple juice, and sea salt in a saucepan and
bring to a boil. Reduce the flame to low, cover, and simmer until the
apples are soft. Dilute the kuzu in a small amount of water and add it to
the cooked fruit, stirring to prevent lumping. Simmer for 2–3 minutes.
Serve over Tofu French Toast (see above) or Mochi Waffles (see below).

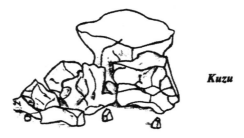

Kuzu

Mochi Waffles

6–8 pieces mochi, 2 inches wide
    by 3 inches long by ¼ inch
    thick

Yield: Six to eight servings.

Place one piece of mochi in each waffle section of your waffle iron. Do
not oil the iron. Cook until the mochi is crisp and slightly browned and
does not stick to the waffle iron. Remove the waffle and repeat until all
the mochi has been used.

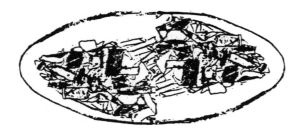

Steamed Collard Greens

4 cups collard greens, washed
  and thinly sliced on a diagonal
water

Yield: Four to five servings.

Place about ¼ inch of water in a saucepan and bring it to a boil. Place the collard greens in the pan, cover, and steam 3–4 minutes, or until the greens start to become tender but still are slightly crisp and bright green in color. Remove them and place them in a serving bowl.

Barley Tea

1 tablespoon roasted barley
1 quart water

Yield: Four to five servings.

Prepackaged, roasted, unhulled barley for making tea can be purchased in most natural food stores. It is sold under the name mugi-cha. You can also make homemade barley tea by roasting barley in a dry skillet over a low flame until it turns golden brown. Stir constantly to evenly roast the barley and prevent burning.

Place the roasted barley in a kettle filled with 1 quart of water. Bring the water to a boil, reduce the flame to low, and simmer to desired strength. For a mild tea try simmering for 3–5 minutes; for a stronger flavor, simmer 10–15 minutes. In the summer months this tea is very refreshing when slightly chilled and served with a slice of lemon on the side.

LIGHT LUNCHES

Noon is often the most busy time of day, in keeping with the daily cycle of energy. Many people prefer a quick, light lunch that doesn't require too much time to prepare or eat. When this is carried to the extreme, however, we may eat on the run without enough care or consideration for our food or its effect on our health. It is important to always keep in mind that food is essential for health and that when we eat, we need to do so in a relaxed and calm manner, chewing each mouthful thoroughly.

The lunch menus in this section are quick and easy to prepare. They are light and enjoyable, and contain a variety of balanced natural dishes. Please enjoy, and don't forget to chew well!

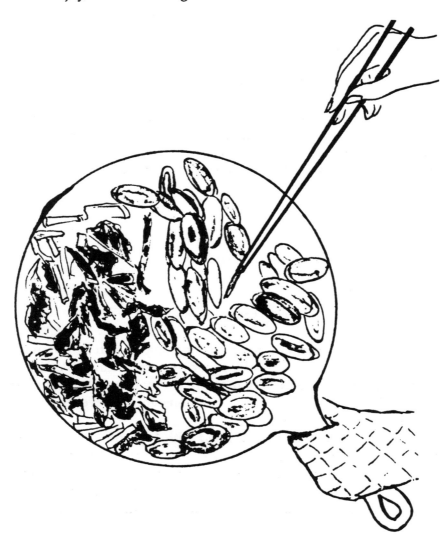

Lunch

Menu One

Fried Rice and Vegetables

Pickled Chinese Cabbage

Boiled Scallions and Dried Tofu

Brown Rice Tea

Fried Rice and Vegetables

> 1 cup onions, sliced into thin
>   half-moons
> 1/4 cup shaved burdock
> 1/2 cup carrots, sliced into thin
>   matchsticks
> 4–5 cups cooked brown rice
> 1/4 cup chopped scallions
> dark sesame oil
> water (optional)
> tamari soy sauce
>
> Yield: Four to five servings.

Place a small amount of dark sesame oil in a skillet and heat it up. Add the onions and sauté 1–2 minutes. Add the burdock and sauté 2–3 minutes. Place the carrots in a layer on top of the onions and burdock, and place the cooked rice on top of the carrots. Do not mix. If the rice is dry, add a few drops of water. Cover the skillet, reduce the flame to low, and simmer until the vegetables are tender. Add a small amount of tamari soy sauce for a mild salt taste. Cover and simmer 3–4 minutes longer. Then place the scallions on top of the rice. Cover and simmer until the scallions are done (1–2 minutes). Mix the rice and vegetables together and place in a serving bowl.

Pickled Chinese Cabbage

4 cups Chinese cabbage, very
    thinly sliced on a diagonal
1/2 teaspoon sea salt

Yield: Four to five servings.

Place the sliced Chinese cabbage in a pickle press and mix in the sea salt
thoroughly. Place the cover on the press and screw it down to apply
pressure. Allow the cabbage to sit for 2–3 hours. If the water level rises
above the pressure plate, release some of the pressure so that the water
level drops just below the plate. After 2-3 hours, remove the pickled
Chinese cabbage; drain and squeeze out excess liquid. If the cabbage
tastes too salty, rinse it quickly under cold water before placing it in a
serving bowl.

Boiled Scallions and Dried Tofu

6–8 pieces of dried tofu, soaked
    and sliced (squeeze out and
    discard the liquid from soaking
    before slicing)
2 bunches of scallions, washed
    and sliced into 2-inch pieces
1/2 teaspoon fresh ginger juice
tamari soy sauce
water

Yield: Four to five servings.

Place the tofu in a saucepan and add water to just cover. Bring to a boil.
Reduce the flame to medium-low, cover, and simmer about 10 minutes.
Add the scallions and ginger juice. Season with a small amount of tamari soy sauce for a mild salt taste. Cover and simmer 1-2 minutes. Remove cover and cook off any remaining liquid. Transfer to a serving
dish.

Brown Rice Tea

½ cup brown rice, washed
1 quart water

Yield: Four to five servings.

Heat up a dry skillet. Place the rice in the skillet and roast it until it turns golden brown, stirring constantly to evenly roast and prevent burning. Remove the rice and place it in a teakettle with 1 quart of water. Bring the water to a boil, reduce the flame to low, and simmer for approximately 15–20 minutes. Strain through a tea strainer and serve hot.

As a variation, try other grains such as barley or hato mugi (unroasted pearl barley), or combine roasted rice with a small amount of bancha twigs (see recipe on page 60). Tea made from brown rice and barley (see page 63) is also very refreshing any time of day.

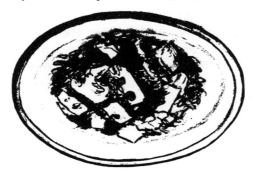

Menu Two

Boiled Fu and Vegetables

Sliced Turnip Greens

Red Radish Pickles

Bancha Tea

Boiled Fu and Vegetables

> 1 package kuruma (round) fu,
>   soaked 5–10 minutes and
>   sliced
> 1 cup fresh green peas
> 1 cup cauliflower flowerettes
> 1/2 cup carrots, sliced into
>   matchsticks
> water
> tamari soy sauce
> sliced scallions
>
> Yield: Four to five servings.

Place the fu in a pot and cover it with water. Bring to a boil. Cover, reduce the flame to medium-low, and simmer about 7–10 minutes. Add the peas, cauliflower, and carrots. Cover and simmer until the vegetables are tender. Season with tamari soy sauce to create a mild salt taste. Simmer 5 minutes longer. Place in individual serving bowls and garnish with sliced scallions.

Sliced Turnip Greens

> 4 cups turnip greens, washed
>   and sliced on a diagonal
> water
>
> Yield: Four to five servings.

Place about 1/4 inch of water in a saucepan and bring it to a boil. Add the turnip greens. Cover and boil 1–2 minutes, until the sliced greens are tender. Remove, drain, and place them in a serving bowl.

Red Radish Pickles

1 bunch red radishes with tops or
    1 package red radishes,
    washed
1/4 cup umeboshi vinegar

Yield: Four to five servings.

Slice the red radishes into thin rounds and place them in a pickle press. Slice the green stems into thin pieces and place them in the press as well. Thoroughly mix in the umeboshi vinegar. Place the top on the pickle press and screw it down to apply pressure. Let the radishes sit for 2–3 hours. After this time, remove them and squeeze out any excess liquid. If the radishes taste too salty, rinse them quickly under cold water first; then squeeze out the excess liquid. Place the pickled radishes in a serving dish.

Bancha Tea

1 tablespoon bancha twigs
1 quart water

Yield: Four to five servings.

For a strong beverage, first place the twigs in a dry stainless steel skillet and roast them for several minutes. For a lighter tea, simply place the twigs in a teakettle without roasting. Add the water and place the kettle over a high flame. Bring to a boil, then reduce the flame to low. For a mild tea, simmer 2–3 minutes. You can simmer the twigs for up to 10 minutes if you prefer strong tea. Serve hot.

Menu Three

Rice Balls

Scrambled Tofu

Steamed Whole Wheat Bread

Boiled Salad

Umeboshi-Sesame-Parsley Dressing

Grain Coffee

Rice Balls

> 2 sheets nori, toasted
> 4–5 cups cooked brown rice
> 2–3 umeboshi plums, broken in
>   half
> water
> pinch of sea salt
>
> Yield: Four to five servings.

Cut each sheet of nori into quarters to obtain 8–12 equal-sized squares. Place a cup of water in a bowl and add a pinch of sea salt. Wet your hands very slightly with the water in the bowl. Pick up 1 cup of cooked brown rice and pack it together (like a snowball) or form it into a triangle by cupping your hands into a "V" shape (as shown in Figure 4.2, following), pressing in from the sides and top. Poke your finger into the center of the rice ball to create a hole and insert between $1/2$–1 umeboshi plum. Reshape the rice ball to cover the hole where the plum was inserted. Then cover one half of the rice ball with a toasted nori square, pressing it so that it sticks firmly. Press another square of toasted nori

Figure 4.2 Making a Rice Ball

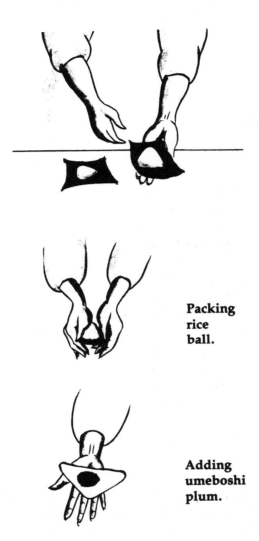

Packing
rice
ball.

Adding
umeboshi
plum.

against the other half of the rice ball to attach it firmly. The rice ball
should now be completely covered with toasted nori.

You may need to wet your hands occasionally to prevent the nori and
rice from sticking to them. It is best to use as little water as possible.
Excess water on your hands when molding and shaping the rice balls
will detract from their taste and appearance. If there are any spots that
are not completely covered with nori, you can patch them by tearing off
small pieces or strips of toasted nori and simply pressing them on the
rice ball as described above, until the rice ball is completely covered.

Repeat the above process until all the rice has been used. The proportions listed above yield 4–5 rice balls. Serve them on an attractive plate or tray.

Scrambled Tofu

$^1/_2$ cup diced onion
$^1/_4$ cup sliced mushrooms
$^1/_4$ cup burdock, sliced into thin
    matchsticks or shaved
$^1/_2$ cup carrots, sliced into thin
    matchsticks
1 cup green beans, thinly sliced
    on a diagonal
$^1/_4$ cup slivered almonds
2 cakes firm-style tofu, drained (2
    pounds of tofu)
$^1/_4$ cup sliced scallions
dark sesame oil
tamari soy sauce

Yield: Four to five servings.

Heat a small amount of dark sesame oil in a skillet. Add the onions and sauté 1–2 minutes. Place the mushrooms in the skillet and sauté 2–3 minutes. Add several drops of tamari soy sauce to brown the mushrooms. Then add the burdock and sauté 2–3 minutes. Next, add the carrots and green beans. Place the slivered almonds on top of the vegetables. Do not mix any of the ingredients. Crumble the tofu on top of the vegetables and cover the skillet. Turn the flame to medium-low and cook until the vegetables are tender and the tofu is soft. Place the scallions on top of the tofu and sprinkle several drops of tamari soy sauce on top to create a mild salt taste. Cover and cook 2–3 minutes, until the scallions are done. Remove the cover and cook off some of the remaining liquid. Mix, place in a serving bowl, and garnish.

Steamed Whole Wheat Bread

6–8 slices whole wheat bread
water

Yield: Four to five servings.

Place about ½ inch of water in a pot and insert a collapsible stainless steel steamer basket. Put the bread in the steamer, cover, and bring the water to a boil. Steam until the bread is soft and moist. Then place it on a serving plate.

Boiled Salad

½ cup daikon, sliced in thick
    rectangles
1 cup broccoli flowerettes
1 cup green cabbage, sliced into
    1-inch squares
¼ cup red onions, sliced into
    thick half-moons
water

Yield: Four to five servings.

Place about ½ inch of water in a pot and bring it to a boil. Add the daikon; cover and boil 1 minute. Carefully remove the daikon and drain it, returning the water to the pot. Add the broccoli. Cover and boil 2–3 minutes, until the broccoli is tender but still slightly crisp and bright green. Remove the broccoli and drain it, again returning the water to the pot. Add the cabbage, cover, and boil 2–3 minutes, until the cabbage starts to become tender but remains slightly crisp. Remove and drain the cabbage and return the water to the pot. Next, place the red onions in the pot. Cover and boil 1–2 minutes. Remove the onions and drain them. Place all the boiled vegetables in a bowl and toss to mix. Either serve the boiled salad with Umeboshi-Sesame-Parsley Dressing (see below) on the side, or mix the dressing in with the vegetables before serving.

Umeboshi-Sesame-Parsley Dressing

2 tablespoons tan sesame seeds,
   roasted
2 umeboshi plums (pits removed)
1 tablespoon chopped or minced
   parsley
water

Yield: Four to five servings.

Grind the sesame seeds in a suribachi until they are about half-crushed.
Remove the seeds and grind the umeboshi plums to a smooth paste.
Add the parsley and grind it together with the plums. Return the
ground sesame seeds to the suribachi. Add enough water to make a
mild salty-sour taste and mix well. Transfer the dressing to a serving
dish and spoon it over boiled salad, or mix it in just before serving.

Grain Coffee

1 teaspoon grain coffee
1 cup boiling water

Yield: One serving.

Instant grain coffee can be found in most natural food stores, but if you
can't locate it, you can prepare your own by individually roasting barley, rice, azuki beans, chickpeas, burdock, or chicory, etc., and grinding
them (again, individually) to a very fine powder in a grain mill. Combine the various ingredients once they have been ground. To prepare
instant grain coffee, put a teaspoonful in a cup and pour boiling water
over it. Stir and drink. Homemade grain coffee can be brewed in a
coffeepot or simmered for several minutes in a saucepan.

Menu Four

Vegetable Fried Udon

Mustard Green Sushi

Pickled Daikon and Lemon Rind

Bancha Tea

Vegetable Fried Udon

1 package (8 ounces) udon
    noodles
1 cup fresh tofu, drained and
    sliced into cubes
1/2 cup carrots, sliced into
    matchsticks
1/2 cup cabbage, thinly sliced on a
    diagonal
1 cup sliced scallions
dark sesame oil
tamari soy sauce
water

Yield: Four to five servings.

Place the udon in 2 quarts of boiling water and stir to prevent lumping. Reduce the flame to medium and simmer, uncovered, several minutes. To test for doneness, break a noodle in half and observe the color. If the inside is still white and the outside light brown, the noodles should cook a little longer. When the inside is the same color as the outside, the noodles are ready. The entire cooking process takes only a few minutes. When the udon is done, place it in a colander or strainer and run cold water over it. Rinsing the noodles prevents them from sticking and removes excess salt. Allow the noodles to drain.

Brush a skillet with a small amount of dark sesame oil and heat it up. Add the tofu and several drops of tamari soy sauce. Sauté 3–5 minutes. Add the carrots and cabbage. Sauté 2–3 minutes. Place the noodles on top of the tofu and vegetables. Cover the skillet and place it over a low flame for several minutes, until the vegetables are tender and the udon is hot. Place the scallions on top of the udon. Add several drops of tamari soy sauce to obtain a mild salt taste. Cover and cook 2–3 minutes, until the scallions are done. Mix and place in a serving dish.

Mustard Green Sushi

1 bunch mustard greens, washed
   and left whole
3–4 sheets toasted nori
¼ cup roasted sesame seeds
several pieces of shiso leaves

Yield: Four to five servings.

Place about ½ inch of water in a pot and bring it to a boil. Place half the bunch of mustard greens in the boiling water, cover, and boil 2–3 minutes, until the leaves are tender but still bright green. Remove the greens, drain, and allow to cool. Cook the remaining greens the same way.

Place a bamboo sushi mat on a cutting board. Set one piece of the toasted nori on top. Divide the mustard greens into 3–4 equal parts and place one part on the toasted nori, close to the bottom edge of the sheet. Sprinkle a teaspoon or so of sesame seeds on top of the mustard greens, covering the entire length of the vegetable. Next, lay 2–3 strips of shiso on top of the mustard greens, forming a line from end to end down the center. Roll the sushi mat up tightly, just as you would for Boiled Chinese Cabbage and Carrot Rolls with Umeboshi Paste (see page 59) and squeeze out any excess liquid. Squeezing out excess liquid will help to seal the nori tightly around the mustard greens. Remove the sushi from the bamboo mat and slice it immediately into 7 or 8 pieces of equal size. Arrange the sushi attractively on a serving platter so that each piece is standing on its end with the mustard greens facing upward.

If you desire, you may make a dip sauce for the sushi, although it is not necessary. Use a small amount of tamari soy sauce, grated ginger, and water.

Pickled Daikon and Lemon Rind

1 piece daikon, 6–8 inches long,
   sliced into rounds ¼-inch thick
1 tablespoon lemon rind, sliced
   into thick matchsticks
½–1 teaspoon sea salt

Yield: Four to five servings.

Slice each round of daikon into thin rectangles. Place the daikon in a pickle press. Add the lemon rind and sea salt. Mix well and place the cover on the press. Screw the cover down to apply pressure and allow the pickle press to sit for 3–4 hours. After this time, remove the lemon rind and discard, rinse the daikon, and place in a serving dish.

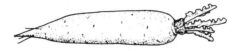

Daikon radish

Bancha Tea

1 tablespoon bancha twigs
1 quart water

Yield: Four to five servings.

For a strong beverage, first place the twigs in a dry stainless steel skillet and roast them for several minutes. For a lighter tea, simply place the twigs in a teakettle without roasting. Add the water and place the kettle over a high flame. Bring to a boil, then reduce the flame to low. For a mild tea, simmer 2–3 minutes. You can simmer the twigs for up to 10 minutes if you prefer strong tea. Serve hot.

Menu Five

Udon and Broth with Fried Tempeh

Daikon and Carrot Pressed Salad

Steamed Broccoli and Cauliflower

Brown Rice and Bancha Tea

Udon and Broth with Fried Tempeh

1 package (8 ounces) udon
   noodles
4–5 cups water
1 strip kombu, 3–4 inches long,
   soaked
4–5 shiitake mushrooms, soaked,
   de-stemmed, and sliced
8 ounces tempeh, cubed and
   deep-fried until golden brown
sliced scallions

Yield: Four to five servings.

Cook the udon noodles and rinse and drain them per the instructions
on package. Set them aside while you prepare the broth.

    Place the water in a pot and add the kombu and shiitake mushrooms.
Cover and bring to a boil. Reduce the flame to medium-low. Simmer 4–
5 minutes; remove the kombu and set it aside for future use. Cover the
pot again and simmer the shiitake for another 5–10 minutes. Season
lightly with tamari soy sauce for a mild salt taste. Place the udon in individual serving bowls and pour the hot broth over them. Garnish each
portion with sliced scallions and several pieces of fried tempeh. Serve
hot.

Daikon and Carrot Pressed Salad

1 cup daikon, sliced into very
    thin matchsticks
1 cup carrots, sliced into very
    thin matchsticks
1/2 teaspoon sea salt
1/4 cup brown rice vinegar
1 tablespoon roasted black
    sesame seeds

Yield: Four to five servings.

Place the daikon, carrot, sea salt, and brown rice vinegar in a pickle press and mix well. Place the cover on top of the press and screw it down to apply pressure. Let the salad sit for 2–3 hours; then remove it and squeeze out excess liquid. If the salad is too salty or sour for your taste, simply rinse it quickly under cold water before placing it in a serving dish. Garnish with a sprinkling of roasted black sesame seeds.

Steamed Broccoli and Cauliflower

2 cups cauliflower flowerettes
2 cups broccoli flowerettes
water

Yield: Four to five servings.

Place about 1/2 inch of water in a pot. Insert a collapsible stainless steel steamer or set a bamboo steamer basket on top of the pot. Place the cauliflower in the steamer. Cover and steam 2–3 minutes, until about half done. Add the broccoli and steam until it is tender but still bright green. Remove the broccoli and cauliflower and place them in a serving bowl.

Brown Rice and Bancha Tea

1 tablespoon bancha twigs
1/4 cup dry-roasted brown rice
1 quart water

Yield: Four to five servings.

Place all ingredients in a kettle and bring to a boil. Reduce the flame to low and simmer about 10 minutes. When serving, strain the tea through a bamboo tea strainer.

Menu Six

Fried Tofu Sandwiches

Hato Mugi Stew

Parsley with Tamari-Ginger Sauce

Bancha Tea

Fried Tofu Sandwiches

6–8 slices tofu
6–8 slices whole wheat bread
6–8 slices of cucumber
1/2 cup sauerkraut
4–5 lettuce leaves, washed
dark sesame oil
tamari soy sauce

Yield: Four to five servings.

Heat a small amount of dark sesame oil in a skillet. Place the tofu in the skillet and sprinkle a couple of drops of tamari soy sauce on each slice.

Fry 3–4 minutes. Flip the tofu over, sprinkle a couple of drops of tamari soy sauce on this side, and fry until browned. Flip the tofu over once more, and fry it for another 2–3 minutes until browned.

Place 2 slices of cucumber, a small amount of sauerkraut, and a couple of lettuce leaves on a slice of bread. Add 2 pieces of fried tofu. Place the top slice of bread on the sandwich. Repeat until you have 3–4 sandwiches. Slice each sandwich in half and place it on an individual serving plate.

Hato Mugi Stew

1 cup hato mugi (pearl barley),
   washed
4–5 shiitake mushrooms, soaked,
   de-stemmed, and diced
1 cup diced celery
½ cup dried daikon, soaked and
   sliced
½ cup diced carrot
1 strip kombu, 3–4 inches long,
   soaked and diced
3–4 cups water
sea salt
sliced scallions

Yield: Four to five servings.

Place the hato mugi, shiitake mushrooms, celery, dried daikon, carrot, and kombu in a pressure cooker. Add the water and a pinch of sea salt. Cover the cooker and bring it up to pressure. Reduce the flame to medium-low and cook for 35 minutes or so. Remove the cooker from the flame, allow the pressure to come down, and remove the cover. Place the cooker back on the flame. Add a small amount of sea salt to create a mild salt taste and simmer for another 10 minutes or so. Place the stew in individual serving bowls and garnish each portion with sliced scallions.

Parsley with Tamari-Ginger Sauce

1 bunch parsley, washed
water
1 teaspoon tamari soy sauce
¼ teaspoon fresh grated ginger
¼ cup water
pinch of sea salt

Yield: Four to five servings.

Place ½ inch of water in a saucepan and bring it to a boil. Add the parsley and sea salt. Cover and boil 1 minute or so. Remove the parsley, drain it, and allow it to cool. Then chop the parsley very fine and place it in a serving dish.

To prepare the sauce, combine the tamari, ginger, and ¼ cup water in a cup. Mix well and heat. Spoon the sauce over the parsley while serving.

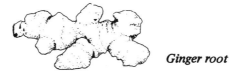

Ginger root

Bancha Tea

1 tablespoon bancha twigs
1 quart water

Yield: Four to five servings.

For a strong beverage, first place the twigs in a dry stainless steel skillet and roast them for several minutes. For a lighter tea, simply place the twigs in a teakettle without roasting. Add the water and place the kettle over a high flame. Bring to a boil, then reduce the flame to low. For a mild tea, simmer 2–3 minutes. You can simmer the twigs for up to 10 minutes if you prefer strong tea. Serve hot.

Menu Seven

Tempeh Sandwiches

Dill Pickles

Sauteed Chinese-Style Vegetables

Barley-Bancha Tea

Tempeh Sandwiches

4–5 squares of tempeh, 3 inches
    by 3 inches by 1/4 inch thick
1/4 teaspoon ginger juice
8–10 slices whole wheat bread
1/2 cup sauerkraut
4–5 lettuce leaves, washed
1/4 cup alfalfa sprouts
tamari soy sauce
water

Yield: Four to five servings.

Place the tempeh in a dry skillet and sprinkle a couple of drops of tamari soy sauce on each side. Heat up the skillet. When it is hot, turn the tempeh slices over and brown. Flip the tempeh over and brown the other side. Add enough water to just cover the tempeh slices. Cover and bring to a boil. Reduce the flame to low, add the ginger juice, and simmer about 20–25 minutes. Turn the flame to high and cook off the remaining liquid. You may add several more drops of tamari soy sauce at this time to obtain a saltier taste, if desired. When all the liquid is gone, brown both sides of the tempeh again. Remove it from the skillet and place it on a plate.

Place a slice of tempeh on a slice of whole wheat bread and garnish it with a tablespoon of sauerkraut, a lettuce leaf or two, and a few sprouts. Place another slice of bread on top to make a sandwich. Slice the sandwich in half and place it on a plate. Prepare the other sandwiches in the same way with the remaining tempeh and bread.

Dill Pickles

> ¼–⅓ cup sea salt
> 8–10 cups water
> 2 pounds fresh pickling
>   cucumbers, quartered
>   lengthwise
> 3–4 sprigs fresh dill
>
> Yield: Four to five servings.

Place the sea salt and water in a pot and bring to a boil. Reduce the flame to low, stir, and simmer until all the salt has dissolved. Remove the pot from the flame and allow the water to cool completely.

Place the sliced cucumbers and dill in a large glass jar and pour the cool brine solution over it until the cucumbers are completely covered. Cover the mouth of the jar with clean cotton cheesecloth and let the cucumbers sit for 3–4 days (2–3 days in warmer weather). Then place the jar in the refrigerator and let it sit for another day or two. The pickles will then be ready to eat. The longer you let them sit, the more salty and sour they become. These pickles will keep for about 5–7 days or more in a cool place.

You may want to try adding other vegetables, such as onion slices, carrot slices, broccoli spears, cauliflower flowerettes, red onion slices, red radishes, or sliced daikon. You may also add a small amount of sauerkraut or brown rice vinegar to the water after it has cooled for a different flavor.

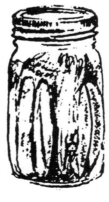

Sautéed Chinese-Style Vegetables

1/2 cup carrots, sliced into
    matchsticks
1 cup Chinese cabbage, thickly
    sliced on a diagonal
1 cup mung bean sprouts,
    washed and drained
1/2 cup snow peas, de-stemmed
dark sesame oil
tamari soy sauce

Yield: Four to five servings.

Place a wok on the burner and brush it with a small amount of oil. Heat up the oil and add the carrots. Sauté over high flame for 1–2 minutes. Add the Chinese cabbage and sauté 1–2 minutes. Add the sprouts and snow peas and sauté until the vegetables are tender but still crisp and brightly colored. Season with a small amount of tamari soy sauce and sauté another minute or so.

For variety, add other vegetables, tofu, seitan, or tempeh. You may also make a sauce, if there is any liquid in the wok, by thickening it with a small amount of diluted kuzu.

Barley-Bancha Tea

1 tablespoon roasted barley
1 tablespoon bancha twigs
1 quart water

Yield: Four to five servings.

Place all the ingredients in a teakettle and bring to a boil. Reduce the flame to low and simmer 5–10 minutes, or until the tea reaches the desired strength. Pour the tea through a strainer when serving.

DELICIOUS DINNERS

As the sun sets in the evening, the earth's atmosphere becomes still and quiet. What a perfect time to enjoy a more elaborate and varied meal in a relaxed and comfortable setting.

Until modern times, dinner gave families the chance to get together to share good food and company. Dinner was most often eaten at home. Today, however, home cooking is disappearing. Americans eat out more now than ever before: one in two meals is eaten away from home, according to surveys. Those who cook for us influence our health and destiny. When we eat out, we are entrusting our health to whoever is in the kitchen. Social occasions may require that we do this now and then, but food that is prepared by someone who has care and concern for our health and well-being is always the best.

The dinners that follow are balanced and complete. They are based on dishes used often macrobiotic cooking, and feature the most basic cooking and cutting methods. We hope you will enjoy preparing and serving them with love and care.

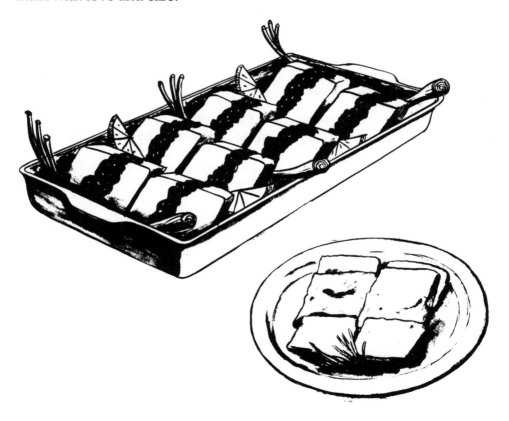

Dinner

Menu One

Pressure-Cooked Brown Rice

Millet Squash Soup

Dried Daikon with Kombu and Shiitake

Chickpeas and Carrots

Steamed Kale

Miso-Scallion Condiment

Apple-Pear Kanten

Bancha Tea

Pressure-Cooked Brown Rice

2 cups organic brown rice,
   washed
$2\frac{1}{2}$–3 cups water
pinch of sea salt per cup of rice

Yield: Four to five servings.

Place the rice and water in a pressure cooker. Set the cooker over a low flame, without the cover, for about 10 minutes. Then add the sea salt, cover, and turn the flame to high. Bring the cooker up to pressure. Reduce the flame to medium-low and place a flame deflector under the cooker. Cook for 50 minutes. After this time, remove the cooker from the flame and allow the pressure to come down. When the pressure is down, remove the cover and let the cooker sit for 4–5 minutes to loosen the rice on the bottom. Remove the rice and place it in a wooden serving bowl. Garnish and serve.

Millet Squash Soup

½ diced onions
½ cup diced celery
1 cup buttercup or butternut
   squash, washed and cubed
¼ cup diced carrots
¼ cup diced burdock
½ cup millet, washed
4–5 cups water
sea salt
choped parsley

Yield: Four to five servings.

Layer the vegetables in a pot in the following order: onions, celery, squash, carrots, and burdock. Place the millet on top of the vegetables. Add enough water to just cover the millet. Add a pinch of sea salt, cover, and bring to a boil. Reduce the flame to medium-low and simmer 30–35 minutes. As the millet expands and absorbs water, add enough only to just cover it. This may need to be done several times during the course of cooking. When the millet is done, you may add enough water to create the desired consistency. Season with a little more sea salt for a mild taste and simmer another 10 minutes or so. Place the soup in individual serving bowls and garnish with chopped parsley.

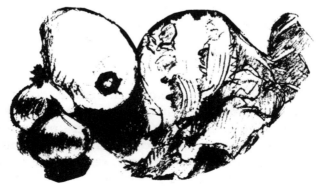

Dried Daikon with Kombu and Shiitake

1 strip kombu, 6–8 inches long,
    soaked and sliced into thin
    matchsticks
4–5 shiitake mushrooms, soaked,
    de-stemmed, and sliced
2 cups dried daikon, washed,
    soaked, and sliced
water from soaking kombu, wa-
    ter from soaking shiitake, and
    water from soaking daikon
tamari soy sauce

Yield: Four to five servings.

Place the kombu and shiitake mushrooms in a skillet. Set the dried daikon on top. Add water to just cover the dried daikon. Cover and bring to a boil. Reduce the flame to low and simmer for 40–45 minutes, until the kombu is soft. Season with a small amount of tamari soy sauce for a mild salt taste and continue to cook until all the remaining liquid is gone. Mix and place in a serving bowl.

Chickpeas and Carrots

1 strip kombu 3–4 inches long,
    soaked and diced
1 cup chickpeas, washed and
    soaked 6–8 hours
1/2 cup carrots, cut into chunks
1/4 cup celery, sliced thickly on a
    diagonal
1/4 cup parsnips, cut into chunks
2 cups water
1/4 teaspoon sea salt

Yield: Four to five servings.

Place the kombu in a pressure cooker and set the chickpeas on top. Add the vegetables and water. Cover and bring to pressure. When the pressure is up, reduce the flame to medium-low and cook for 1–1 1/4 hours.

Remove the cooker from the flame and allow the pressure to come down. Then remove the cover and add the sea salt. Place the pressure cooker back over the flame (without the cover) and simmer another 10–15 minutes. Place the chickpeas and carrots in a serving bowl.

Steamed Kale

4 cups kale, washed and sliced
    on a diagonal
water

Yield: Four to five servings.

Place ½ inch of water in a pot and either set a stainless steel steamer basket inside or a bamboo steamer on top of the pot. Bring the water to a boil. Place the kale in the steamer, cover, and steam until it is tender but still slightly crisp and bright green. Remove the kale and place it in a serving bowl.

Miso-Scallion Condiment

1 bunch scallions with roots,
    washed
2–3 tablespoons puréed barley
    miso
dark sesame oil
water

Yield: Four to five servings.

Make sure the scallions are cleaned well with a vegetable brush to remove soil. Finely mince the scallion roots. Brush a small amount of dark sesame oil in a skillet and heat it up. Add the minced scallion roots and sauté 1 minute or so. Chop the green and white part of the scallion and add this to the skillet. Sauté another minute or so. Make a little hole in the center of scallions and place the puréed miso in it. Add a teaspoon or so of water, cover, and bring to a boil. Reduce the flame to low and simmer 5–7 minutes. Remove the cover, mix, and cook any remaining liquid off. Place the condiment in a serving dish; use it for rice or other grains.

Apple-Pear Kanten

1 cup apples, washed, peeled,
  and sliced
1 cup pears, washed, peeled, and
  sliced
1/2 cup raisins
2 cups apple juice
2 cups water
pinch of sea salt
agar-agar flakes (read directions
  on the package for correct
  amount of agar for 4 cups of
  liquid)

Yield: Four to five servings.

Place all of the ingredients in a pot over a high flame. Stir several times to help the agar flakes dissolve. Bring to a boil, reduce the flame to low, and simmer 2–3 minutes. Remove the mixture and pour it into a bowl. Set it in a cool place until jelled. Slice the kanten scoop it out and serve it in individual dessert cups.

Bancha Tea

1 tablespoon bancha twigs
1 quart water

Yield: Four to five servings.

For a strong beverage, first place the twigs in a dry stainless steel skillet and roast them for several minutes. For a lighter tea, simply place the twigs in a teakettle without roasting. Add the water and place the kettle over a high flame. Bring to a boil, then reduce the flame to low. For a mild tea, simmer 2–3 minutes. You can simmer the twigs for up to 10 minutes if you prefer strong tea. Serve hot.

Menu Two

Sweet Rice and Azuki Beans

Vegetable Soup

Arame with Lotus Root and Onions

Pressed Salad

Steamed Broccoli with Tofu Cream Dressing

Barley Tea

Sweet Rice and Azuki Beans

2/3 cup azuki beans, washed
2¹/2–3 cups water (including the
    water from cooking the azuki
    beans)
1¹/3 cups sweet brown rice,
    washed
pinch of sea salt per cup of rice
    and beans

Yield: Four to five servings.

Place the azuki beans in a saucepan and cover them with water. Bring to a boil. Reduce the flame to medium-low and simmer the beans for about 20 minutes. Remove them from the flame and pour the cooking water into a measuring cup. Add enough plain water to the measuring cup to equal 2¹/2–3 cups.

Mix together the sweet rice and the azuki beans in a pressure cooker. Add the water and sea salt. Cover the cooker and bring it up to pressure. Reduce the flame to medium-low and place a flame deflector under the cooker. Cook for 50 minutes. After this time, remove the cooker from the flame and allow the pressure to come down. Let the rice and beans sit in the uncovered pressure cooker for 4–5 minutes before placing them in a wooden serving bowl.

Vegetable Soup

4–5 cups water
1 strip kombu, 3–4 inches long,
    soaked and sliced into thin
    matchsticks
4–5 shiitake mushrooms, soaked,
    de-stemmed, and sliced
1 cup carrots, sliced in
    matchsticks
1/2 cup daikon, thinly sliced into
    rectangles
1/2 cup yellow waxed beans,
    sliced diagonally into long,
    thin pieces
1 cup scallions, sliced in 2-inch
    lengths
4–5 teaspoons kuzu, diluted in a
    small amount of water
sea salt

Yield: Four to five servings.

Place the water in a pot and add the kombu and shiitake. Cover and bring to a boil. Reduce the flame to medium-low and simmer about 10 minutes. Add the carrots, daikon, and yellow waxed beans. Cover and simmer until the vegetables are tender. Add the scallions, cover, and simmer for half a minute. Add the kuzu, stirring constantly to prevent lumping. Add enough sea salt to obtain a mild salt taste. Simmer the soup 4–5 minutes, then place it in individual serving bowls. Garnish each serving with sprig of watercress or parsley.

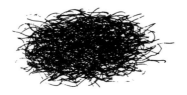

Arame

Arame with Lotus Root and Onions

$^{1}/_{2}$ cup onions, sliced in thin
  half-moons
1 cup lotus root (sliced fresh or
  dried), soaked
1 ounce arame ($1^{1}/_{2}$–2 cups),
  rinsed, drained, and sliced
dark sesame oil
water
tamari soy sauce

Yield: Four to five servings.

Brush a small amount of sesame oil in a skillet and heat it up. Add the onions and saute 2–3 minutes or until they become translucent. Add the lotus root. Set the arame on top of the lotus root. Add enough water to just cover the vegetables. Add 2 drops of tamari soy sauce, cover the skillet, and bring the water to a boil. Reduce the flame to medium-low and simmer 25–30 minutes. Season with a small amount of tamari soy sauce for a mild salt taste and simmer, uncovered, until all the remaining liquid is gone. Mix and place in a serving bowl. Garnish with a sprig of parsley, and serve.

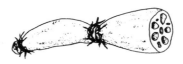

Lotus root

Pressed Salad

1 cup lettuce, washed and thinly
   sliced
1/4 cup celery, thinly sliced on a
   diagonal
1/4 cup onion, sliced into thin
   rounds
1/4 cup red radish, sliced into thin
   rounds
1/4 cup cucumber, sliced on a diagonal and then into
   matchsticks
1/2 teaspoon sea salt
1/4 cup brown rice vinegar

Yield: Four to five servings.

Place all the ingredients in a pickle press and mix them thoroughly.
Place the cover on the press and screw it down to apply pressure. Let
the press sit for 2–3 hours. Remove the vegetables, squeeze out excess
liquid, and place the salad in a serving bowl. If it is too salty, rinse it
quickly under cold water before serving.

Steamed Broccoli with Tofu Cream Dressing

1 cake tofu (1 pound of tofu)
3 umeboshi plums, pitted
1 small onion, finely grated
1/2 teaspoon tamari soy sauce
1/2 cup water
4 cups steamed broccoli

Yield: Four to five servings.

Place the tofu in a hand food mill and purée until it becomes smooth. In
a suribachi, purée the umeboshi plums to obtain a smooth paste. Add
the grated onion, the tofu, and the tamari soy sauce. Purée until the
dressing is smooth and mixed thoroughly. Add a small amount of water
to obtain the desired consistency. Place the broccoli in a serving bowl.
You may mix the tofu dressing in with the broccoli before serving or

place a tablespoon or so of dressing on top of each portion when serving.

Barley Tea

1 tablespoon roasted barley
1 quart water

Yield: Four to five servings.

Prepackaged, roasted, unhulled barley for making tea can be purchased in most natural food stores. It is sold under the name mugi-cha. You can also make homemade barley tea by roasting barley in a dry skillet over a low flame until it turns golden brown. Stir constantly to evenly roast the barley and prevent burning.

Place the roasted barley in a kettle filled with 1 quart of water. Bring the water to a boil, reduce the flame to low, and simmer to desired strength. For a mild tea try simmering for 3–5 minutes; for a stronger flavor, simmer 10–15 minutes. In the summer months this tea is very refreshing when slightly chilled and served with a slice of lemon on the side.

Menu Three

Gomoku

French Onion Soup

Boiled Turnip Greens

Nori Condiment

Red Radishes and Kuzu Sauce

Apple Crunch

Bancha Tea

Gomoku

2 cups organic brown rice, dry-
roasted until golden brown

3 pieces dried tofu, soaked and
diced

¼ cup dried daikon, soaked and
sliced

¼ cup lotus seeds, soaked 2–3
hours

4 shiitake mushrooms, soaked,
de-stemmed, and diced

1 strip kombu, 3–4 inches long,
soaked and diced

½ cup diced carrots

½ cup diced seitan

1 tablespoon minced burdock

2½–3 cups water

Yield: Four to five servings.

Place all of the ingredients in a pressure cooker and mix them well.
Place the cover on the pressure cooker and bring it up to pressure. Reduce the flame to medium-low, place a flame deflector under the
cooker, and pressure cook for 45–50 minutes. Then remove the cooker
from the flame and allow the pressure to come down. Remove the cover
and let the rice sit for 4–5 minutes. Transfer it to a wooden serving
bowl.

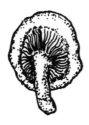 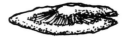

Shiitake mushroom, dried

French Onion Soup

5 cups onions, sliced in thin
   half-moons
4–5 cups water
1 strip kombu, 3–4 inches long,
   soaked and sliced into
   matchsticks
4–5 shiitake mushrooms, soaked,
   de-stemmed, and sliced
dark sesame oil (optional)
tamari soy sauce (or puréed
   barley miso)
pinch of sea salt
sliced scallions

Yield: Four to five servings.

Brush a small amount of oil in a pot and heat it up. Add the onions and
sauté them for 4–5 minutes or until they become translucent. Add the
water, kombu, sea salt, and shiitake mushrooms. Cover and bring to a
boil. Reduce the flame to medium-low and simmer 25–30 minutes so
that the onions get very soft. Season with tamari soy sauce for a mild
salt taste. Simmer 5–10 minutes longer. Place the soup in individual
serving bowls and garnish with sliced scallions.

   For variety, toasted mochi, deep-fried whole wheat bread cubes, or
dry-roasted tamari-seasoned bread cubes may be used in addition to the
scallion garnish. Puréed barley miso may be substitued for tamari soy
sauce to create a different flavor.

Boiled Turnip Greens

1 bunch turnip greens (4–5 cups),
   washed and left whole
water

Yield: Four to five servings.

Place 1/2 inch of water in a pot and bring it to a boil. Place the whole
turnip leaves in the boiling water. Cover and simmer 2–3 minutes. Re-

move the greens, drain, and allow to cool. Slice them into 1-inch lengths and place them in a serving dish.

Nori Condiment

5 sheets nori (untoasted)
water
tamari soy sauce

Yield: Four to five servings.

Tear the nori into small pieces and place them in a saucepan. Add enough water to just cover the nori. Cover the saucepan and bring the water to a boil. Reduce the flame to low and simmer 10 minutes, until the nori becomes very soft. Season with several drops of tamari soy sauce for a mild salt taste. Simmer, uncovered, 2–5 minutes longer, or until almost all of the remaining liquid is gone. Place the condiment in a serving bowl and use it in small amounts with grain dishes.

Red Radishes and Kuzu Sauce

1–2 tablespoons whole shiso
    leaves
1 cup red radishes, washed, and
    with stems and roots removed
2 cups water
2–3 heaping teaspoons kuzu,
    diluted in a small amount of
    water
1 tablespoon chopped parsley

Yield: Four to five servings.

Place the shiso leaves and radishes in a saucepan. Add water, cover, and bring to a boil. Reduce the flame to medium-low and simmer until the radishes are tender. Remove the shiso leaves and set them aside, leaving the cooking water in the pot. Remove the radishes and place them in a serving bowl, again leaving the water in the pot. Chop the shiso very fine and place them in the center of the radishes. Add the diluted kuzu to the cooking water, stirring constantly to prevent lumping. When the liquid becomes thick, simmer 1 minute; then pour the sauce over the radishes. Sprinkle chopped parsley on top for a garnish, and serve.

Apple Crunch

4–5 apples, washed, cored, and
  sliced
1 cup apple juice
1 tablespoon arrowroot flour,
  diluted in 2 tablespoons of
  water
pinch of sea salt

Yield: Four to five servings.

Crunch

1/2 cup rolled oats, dry-roasted
  until golden brown
1/4 cup walnuts, dry-roasted and
  chopped
1/4 cup almonds, dry-roasted and
  chopped
1 tablespoon filberts, dry-roasted
  and chopped
1/4 cup rice syrup or barley malt

Place the apples, sea salt, and juice in a saucepan. Cover and bring to a boil. Reduce the flame to low and simmer until the apples are soft and tender. Add the dissolved arrowroot flour, stirring constantly to prevent lumping. Simmer 1–2 minutes longer. Remove the apples and place them in a baking dish.

Combine all the ingredients for the crunch and mix them together thoroughly. Sprinkle the crunch on top of the apples. Place the baking dish in a 350 F oven and bake until the topping is golden brown and crisp. Remove the apple crunch, allow it to cool, and serve.

Bancha Tea

1 tablespoon bancha twigs
1 quart water

Yield: Four to five servings.

For a strong beverage, first place the twigs in a dry stainless steel skillet and roast them for several minutes. For a lighter tea, simply place the twigs in a teakettle without roasting. Add the water and place the kettle over a high flame. Bring to a boil, then reduce the flame to low. For a mild tea, simmer 2–3 minutes. You can simmer the twigs for up to 10 minutes if you prefer strong tea. Serve hot.

Menu Four

Brown Rice and Barley

Puréed Squash Soup

Japanese Black Soybeans

Nishime Vegetables

Onion Pickles

Boiled Kale with Miso-Walnut Dressing

Bancha Tea

Brown Rice and Barley

1½ cup organic brown rice,
   washed
½ cup barley, washed
2½–3 cups water
pinch of sea salt per cup of grain

Yield: Four to five servings.

Place the brown rice, barley, and water in a pressure cooker and let the grains soak for 6–8 hours. Add the sea salt, cover the pressure cooker and bring it up to pressure. Reduce the flame to medium-low and place a flame deflector under the cooker. Pressure cook for 50 minutes. Then remove the cooker from the flame and allow the pressure to come down. Remove the cover and let the grain sit for 4–5 minutes before removing it and placing it in a wooden serving bowl.

Puréed Squash Soup

5 cups cubed buttercup squash
   or Hokkaido pumpkin,
   skin removed
4–5 cups water
¼–½ teaspoon sea salt
sliced scallions

Yield: Four to five servings.

Place the squash, the water, and only a pinch of the sea salt in a pot. Cover and bring to a boil. Reduce the flame to low and simmer until the squash is very soft. Remove the squash from the flame and purée it in a hand food mill. Pour the puréed squash into the pot, add the remaining sea salt, and return the pot to the flame. Simmer over a low flame for another 10 minutes. Place in individual serving bowls and garnish with sliced scallions.

Japanese Black Soybeans

2 cups Japanese black soybeans
6 cups water
$^1/_4$–$^1/_2$ teaspoon sea salt
1$^1/_4$–1$^1/_2$ tablespoons tamari soy
    sauce

Yield: Four to five servings.

Wash these beans differently from other beans, as their skins become loose if they are washed in water. To wash them, simply dampen a clean kitchen towel and place the beans on the towel. Fold all four sides of the towel over the beans to completely cover them. Roll or knead the beans for about one minute inside the towel. Remove the beans, rinse the towel, and squeeze it out. Repeat rolling the beans in the towel 1–2 more times.

After you clean the beans, place them in a glass or ceramic bowl and add about 6 cups of water and the sea salt. If you omit soaking the beans in salt water, the skins may fall off. For best results, soak the beans 6–8 hours or overnight.

Place the beans and the salted soaking water in a pot and bring to a boil. Do not cover the pot. Reduce the flame to medium-low and simmer until the beans are about 90 percent done. While they are cooking, a gray foam will float to the surface of the water. Skim this off and discard it. Also, during cooking you may need to add small amounts of water from time to time as the water evaporates and the beans expand and absorb it. When the beans are about 90 percent done, add the tamari soy sauce and shake the pot very gently up and down to evenly coat the beans with the liquid. Do not stir or mix with a spoon, however, as the beans are very easily damaged. Cook until almost all of the remaining liquid is gone and the beans are soft and tender. The total cooking time for these beans is approximately 3–3$^1/_2$ hours.

Note: Do not pressure cook Japanese black soybeans if they have been soaked in the above manner, as the skins may clog the pressure gauge. When you combine these beans with rice they can be pressure cooked as long as you wash and dry-roast them first.

Nishime Vegetables

1 strip kombu, 6–8 inches long,
    soaked and sliced into 1/4 inch
    wide strips
4–5 shiitake mushrooms, soaked,
    de-stemmed, and halved
4–5 pieces tofu, 3 inches long by
    2 inches wide by 1/2 inch thick,
    deep-fried or pan-fried until
    golden brown
1/2 cup burdock, thickly sliced on
    a diagonal
3 round slices of fresh lotus root,
    1/4 inch thick, cut in half
3 round slices of daikon, 1/2 inch
    thick, cut in half
pinch of sea salt
water
tamari soy sauce
chopped parsley

Yield: Four to five servings.

Place the kombu in the bottom of a pot. Set the shiitake mushrooms on top of the kombu. Next, layer the fried tofu, the burdock, the lotus root, and finally the daikon on top of the kombu. (If you prefer, you may place the burdock closer to the bottom of the pot so that it will become softer.) Add about 1/2 inch of water and a small pinch of sea salt. Cover the pot and bring the water to a boil. Reduce the flame to low and simmer 30–35 minutes, until the vegetables are soft and tender. Add a small amount of tamari soy sauce for a mild salt taste and simmer until almost all of the remaining liquid is gone. Remove the cover and mix the vegetables to evenly coat them with the sweet cooking water and continue to cook for another minute or so—until all the liquid is gone. Place the vegetables in a serving bowl and garnish with chopped parsley.

Onion Pickles

2 cups onions, sliced in thin
   half-moons
2 tablespoons tamari soy sauce
2 teaspoons brown rice vinegar
water

Yield: Four to five servings.

Place about ½ inch of water in a saucepan and bring to a boil. Add the onions and blanch them for 1 minute. Drain the onions and allow them to cool; then place them in a pickle press. Mix in the tamari soy sauce and brown rice vinegar. Put the cover on the pickle press and screw it down to apply pressure. Let the onions sit for 2–3 hours. Then remove them, rinse, and place them in a serving dish.

Boiled Kale with Miso-Walnut Dressing

1 small bunch kale, washed
3 tablespoons walnuts, dry-
   roasted and chopped fine
2 tablespoons puréed barley miso
1–2 teaspoons lemon juice
½–¾ cup water

Yield: Four to five servings.

Boil or steam the bunch of kale, leaving it whole. Allow it to cool and drain before slicing. To make the Miso Walnut Dressing, place the walnuts in a suribachi and grind them finely but not to a paste. Add the miso and grind some more. Add the lemon juice and mix; add water to taste and mix again. Serve the dressing over the boiled kale (or, for variety, over other vegetables).

Bancha Tea

1 tablespoon bancha twigs
1 quart water

Yield: Four to five servings.

For a strong beverage, first place the twigs in a dry stainless steel skillet
and roast them for several minutes. For a lighter tea, simply place the
twigs in a teakettle without roasting. Add the water and place the kettle
over a high flame. Bring to a boil, then reduce the flame to low. For a
mild tea, simmer 2–3 minutes. You can simmer the twigs for up to 10
minutes if you prefer strong tea. Serve hot.

Menu Five

Brown Rice and Wheat Berries

Soybean Stew

Sweet Sea Palm

Kinpira Burdock with Sesame-Vinegar Dressing

Chinese Cabbage and Watercress Rolls

Applesauce

Barley Tea

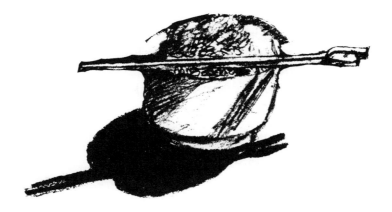

Brown Rice and Wheat Berries

1½ cups organic brown rice,
   washed
½ cup whole wheat berries,
   soaked 6–8 hours
2½–3 cups water
pinch of sea salt per cup of grain

Yield: Four to five servings.

Place the brown rice, whole wheat berries, and water in a pressure cooker and place the cooker, uncoverd, over a low flame for about 10 minutes. Add the sea salt and cover. Bring the cooker up to pressure, reduce the flame to medium-low, and place a flame deflector under the cooker. Cook for 50 minutes. Then remove the cooker from the flame and allow the pressure to come down. Take off the cover and let the food sit for 4–5 minutes. Then remove the rice and wheat and place it in a wooden serving bowl.

Soybean Stew

1 cup white soybeans, washed
  and soaked 6–8 hours
1 strip kombu, 4–5 inches long,
  soaked and diced
2 shiitake mushrooms, soaked,
  de-stemmed, and diced
1/4 cup dried daikon, rinsed,
  soaked, and sliced
1/4 cup dried tofu, soaked and
  cubed
1/4 cup celery, thickly sliced on a
  diagonal
1/2 cup carrots, cut into chunks
2 tablespoons burdock, sliced
  into thick quarters
1/4 cup dried lotus root, soaked
  and sliced
4–5 cups water (Include the water from the soaking the
  kombu, shiitake, daikon, and
  lotus root. Do not use the water from soaking the dried
  tofu.)
tamari soy sauce
grated ginger
sliced scallions

Yield: Four to five servings.

Place all the ingredients except the tamari soy sauce, grated ginger, and
scallions in a pressure cooker. Cover and bring the cooker up to pressure. Reduce the flame to medium-low and cook for 50 minutes. After
this time, remove the cooker from the flame and allow the pressure to
come down. Remove the cover and place the cooker back on the flame.
Season with tamari soy sauce for a mild salt taste and simmer another
10 minutes. Place the stew in individual serving bowls and garnish each
bowl with a dab of grated ginger and a few sliced scallions. Serve hot.

Sweet Sea Palm

2 cups sea palm, soaked and
  sliced
2 tablespoons mirin
water
tamari soy sauce

Yield: Four to five servings.

Place the sea palm in a saucepan. Add enough water to just cover.
Cover the saucepan and bring the water to a boil. Reduce the flame to
medium-low and cook for 25–30 minutes, until the sea palm becomes
tender. Add the mirin and a small amount of tamari soy sauce to create
a mild salt taste. Continue to cook until all the remaining liquid is gone.
Remove the sea palm and place it in a serving dish.

Kinpira Burdock with Sesame-Vinegar Dressing

dark sesame oil
3 cups shaved burdock
water
tamari soy sauce
1/4 cup tan sesame seeds, roasted
1 tablespoon brown rice vinegar
1/4 cup water

Kinpira is a method of cooking in which vegetables are cut finely and
sautéed in sesame oil or with water, and seasoned lightly with tamari
soy sauce.
   To prepare these kinpira vegetables, brush a small amount of dark
sesame oil in a skillet and heat it up. Add the burdock and sauté 2–3
minutes. Add just enough water to cover the bottom of the skillet.
Cover and bring to a boil. Reduce the flame to low and simmer until the
burdock is tender. Season with a small amount of tamari soy sauce for a
mild salt taste and continue to cook until all the remaining liquid is
gone.
   To prepare the dressing, place the roasted sesame seeds in a suribachi
and grind until the seeds are about half-crushed. Add the vinegar and
water. Mix well. Place the sautéed burdock in the suribachi and mix
well to coat it with the dressing. Transfer it to a serving dish.

As a variation, instead of sautéing the burdock, boil it in a mixture of water and vinegar. Then prepare the dressing as described above, adding a few drops of tamari soy sauce.

Chinese Cabbage and Watercress Rolls

9-12 medium-large Chinese
   cabbage leaves
2 bunches watercress
1 teaspoon umeboshi paste
water

Yield: Four to five servings.

Place about 1 inch of water in a pot and bring it to a boil. Place the Chinese cabbage leaves in the pot and cover. Boil the Chinese cabbage 2-3 minutes, until it is basically tender, but still firm and slightly crisp.

Carefully remove the Chinese cabbage and spread it out in a colander to drain and cool. Place watercress in the same boiling water, cover, and boil 1 minute. Remove the watercress, rinse quickly under cold water, and drain.

To assemble the sushi, refer to diagram on page 59. Place a bamboo sushi mat on a cutting board. Place 2 cabbage leaves across the length of the mat in alternate directions, with the hard stem parts facing out toward sides of the mat. Then take 2 more leaves and place them on top of the first leaves so that they cover about half of the bottom layer of the original leaves. Place 1 layer of watercress in the center of leaves, so that it spans the entire length of the leaves.

Pull up the sushi mat slightly with your fingers and press firmly against the cabbage leaves. Hold the mat with your thumbs and index fingers. With your other fingers, tuck the cabbage leaves under as you roll them up. Continue to roll up the sushi mat, pressing firmly to produce a tightly rolled cylinder of leaves. When the leaves are completely rolled into a cylinder, wrap the sushi mat around them tightly and firmly squeeze the roll to remove any excess liquid.

Remove the sushi mat and place the cabbage roll on a cutting board. With a sharp knife, slice the cabbage roll in half. Then slice each half into 4 equal-sized pieces about 1 inch long. Stand each slice on end on a serving platter so that the watercress is displayed in the center. Place a small dab of umeboshi paste on top of each piece. Repeat with the remaining cabbage leaves and watercress.

For variety, other large leafy greens, such as kale, collards, chard, or mustard greens can be rolled in the same way. Carrot is used in a variation of this recipe on page 58.

Applesauce

8–10 apples, washed, peeled,
   and sliced
pinch of sea salt
1 cup water

Yield: Four to five servings.

Place all of the ingredients in a saucepan, cover, and bring to a boil. Reduce the flame to low and simmer until the apples are soft. Purée the apples in a hand food mill. Then place the applesauce in individual serving dishes. Garnish each portion with a few raisins or roasted chopped nuts.

Barley Tea

1 tablespoon roasted barley
1 quart water

Yield: Four to five servings.

Prepackaged, roasted, unhulled barley for making tea can be purchased in most natural food stores. It is sold under the name mugi-cha. You can also make homemade barley tea by roasting barley in a dry skillet over a low flame until it turns golden brown. Stir constantly to evenly roast the barley and prevent burning.

Place the roasted barley in a kettle filled with 1 quart of water. Bring the water to a boil, reduce the flame to low, and simmer to desired strength. For a mild tea try simmering for 3–5 minutes; for a stronger flavor, simmer 10–15 minutes.

In the summer months this tea is very refreshing when slightly chilled and served with a slice of lemon on the side.

Menu Six

Millet and Sweet Corn

Puréed Cauliflower Soup

Sweet and Sour Seitan

Boiled Watercress

Shio Kombu

Glazed Apples

Brown Rice Tea

Millet and Sweet Corn

2 cups millet, washed
1 cup sweet corn
2½ cups water
pinch of sea salt

Yield: Four to five servings.

Heat a skillet and dry-roast the millet until it turns golden brown.
Transfer the millet to a pressure cooker. Add the sweet corn, water, and
sea salt. Cover the cooker and bring it up to pressure. Reduce the flame
to medium-low and cook for 15 minutes. Remove the cooker from the
flame and allow the pressure to come down. Then take off the cover
and let the grain sit for 4–5 minutes. Place it in a wooden serving bowl,
garnish, and serve.

Puréed Cauliflower Soup

5 cups cauliflower flowerettes
    (about 1 large head of
    cauliflower)
4–5 cups water
sea salt
lemon slices, cut in half-moons
chopped parsley

Yield: Four to five servings.

Place the cauliflower, water, and a pinch of sea salt in a pot; cover and bring to a boil. Reduce the flame to low and simmer until the cauliflower is very soft. Remove the cauliflower with the cooking water and purée it in a hand food mill. Then place the purée back in the pot and add a small amount of sea salt to obtain a mild salt taste. Cook for another 10 minutes. Place the soup in individual serving bowls. Garnish each bowl with a half-slice of lemon and a little bit of chopped parsley.

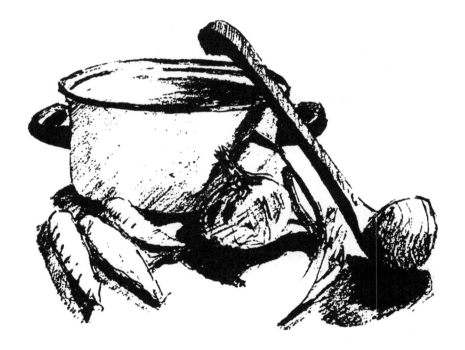

Sweet and Sour Seitan

3 cups cooked seitan, sliced
1 cup apple juice
2 cups water
1 cup onions, sliced in ¼ inch
   thick rounds or rings
½ cup carrots, sliced into thick
   matchsticks
¼ cup celery, thickly sliced on
   diagonal
¼ cup summer squash, sliced on
   a diagonal and then sliced in
   half
3–4 tablespoons kuzu, dissolved
   in 3–4 tablespoons of water
¼ cup sliced scallions
brown rice vinegar
tamari soy sauce

Yield: Four to five servings.

Place the seitan, apple juice, and water in a pot. Cover and bring to a boil. Reduce the flame to medium-low and simmer about 10 minutes. Add the onions, carrots, celery, and summer squash. Simmer until the vegetables are tender. Reduce the flame to low and add a small amount of brown rice vinegar and the diluted kuzu, stirring constantly until the mixture thickens. Season with a small amount of tamari soy sauce to create a mild salt taste, and simmer 5–7 minutes more. Place the sweet and sour seitan in a serving bowl. Garnish with sliced scallions and serve.

Boiled Watercress

2 bunches watercress, washed
water

Yield: Four to five servings.

Place about 2 inches of water in a pot and bring it to a boil. Add half of the watercress, cover, and bring to a boil again. Boil about 30–40 seconds. Remove the watercress, drain it, and allow it to cool. Repeat with the remaining half of the watercress. Serve it whole or slice it into 1/2-inch pieces.

Shio Kombu

2 strips kombu, 10–12 inches
    long, soaked and cubed
water
tamari soy sauce

Yield: Four to five servings.

Place the kombu in a pot and just cover with a mixture of 2/3 water and 1/3 tamari soy sauce, or, if you prefer a saltier taste, half water and half tamari soy sauce. Bring to a boil, cover, and reduce the flame to medium low. Simmer until the kombu is soft. Remove the cover and simmer until almost all liquid is gone. Since shio kombu is salty, only 2-3 one-inch squares should be eaten at a time.

Glazed Apples

4–5 organic or unwaxed baking
    apples, washed and cored
1/2 cup water
1 teaspoon kuzu, diluted in 1–2
    teaspoons water
pinch of sea salt

Yield: Four to five servings.

Place the cored apples in a baking dish. Add the water and cover. Bake at 350°F for 25–30 minutes or until the apples are soft but not split. Gently remove the apples and place them in a serving dish. Place the sweet cooking water in a saucepan and add the diluted kuzu and sea salt. Stirring constantly to prevent lumping, bring the liquid to a boil. Reduce the flame to low and simmer 1–2 minutes. Pour the glaze over the apples and serve.

Brown Rice Tea

¹/₂ cup brown rice, washed
1 quart water

Yield: Four to five servings.

Heat up a dry skillet. Place the rice in the skillet and roast it until it turns golden brown, stirring constantly to evenly roast and prevent burning. Remove the rice and place it in a teakettle with 1 quart of water. Bring the water to a boil, reduce the flame to low, and simmer to approximately 15–20 minutes. Strain through a tea strainer and serve hot.

As a variation, try other grains such as barley or hato mugi (unroasted pearl barley), or combine roasted rice with a small amount of bancha twigs (see recipe on page 60). Tea made from brown rice and barley (see page 63) is also very refreshing any time of day.

Menu Seven

Brown Rice and Shiso Leaves

Clear Soup with Vegetables

Broiled Filet of Sole

Grated Daikon

Hiziki with Sweet Corn and Green Beans

Boiled Kale and Carrots

Amazake Peach Pudding

Bancha Tea

Brown Rice and Shiso Leaves

2 cups organic brown rice,
    washed
2¹/₂–3 cups water
pinch of sea salt per cup of grain
1¹/₄ tablespoons finely minced
    shiso leaves

Yield: Four to five servings.

Place the brown rice, water, and sea salt in a pressure cooker. Cover the cooker, turn the flame to high, and bring the cooker up to pressure. Reduce the flame to medium-low and place a flame deflector under the cooker. Cook for 50 minutes, then remove the cooker from the flame and allow the pressure to come down. Remove the cover and let the rice sit for 4–5 minutes. Transfer the rice to a serving bowl one spoonful at a time, and gradually add the shiso leaves, mixing them in thoroughly with the rice as it is removed.

Clear Soup with Vegetables

4–5 cups water
1 strip kombu, 4–5 inches long,
    soaked
1 cup Chinese cabbage, sliced on
    a diagonal
¹/₂ cup carrots, sliced in flower
    shapes
¹/₂ cup turnips, washed, peeled,
    and cubed
tamari soy sauce
sliced scallions

Yield: Four to five servings.

Place the water and kombu in a pot, cover, and bring to a boil. Reduce the flame to medium-low and simmer 5–7 minutes. Remove the kombu and set it aside for future use. Add the carrots and turnips. Cover and simmer until tender. Add the Chinese cabbage. Reduce the flame to low, season with a little tamari soy sauce (to taste), cover, and simmer

3–4 minutes more. Place the broth in individual serving bowls and garnish each portion with sliced scallions.

Broiled Filet of Sole

> ¼ cup tamari soy sauce
> ¼ cup mirin
> 1 teaspoon fresh grated ginger
> 1–1½ pounds sole, washed
>
> Yield: Four to five servings.

Mix the tamari, mirin, and ginger together in a cup and pour the mixture over the sole. Let the fish marinate for about ½–1 hour. Then transfer it to a baking sheet. Place it under the broiler and broil several minutes, until it is tender and slightly browned. Place the broiled sole on a serving platter and garnish with sprigs of parsley and several slices of lemon. Serve with grated daikon.

Grated Daikon

> 1 piece daikon root, 4–6 inches
>   long, washed
> tamari soy sauce
>
> Yield: Four to five servings.

Grate the daikon on a flat grater and place it in a small dish (there will be about ½ cup). Garnish with several drops of tamari soy sauce and a few scallion slices. Eat grated daikon with mochi (or with seafood or fried dishes) to aid digestion.

Hiziki with Sweet Corn and Green Beans

1 ounce hiziki, washed, soaked,
   and sliced (about 1 ½–2 cups
   soaked)
1 cup green beans, thinly sliced
   on a diagonal
1 cup sweet corn
water
tamari soy sauce
dark sesame oil

Yield: Four to five servings.

Heat a small amount of dark sesame oil in a skillet. Add the hiziki and sauté 1–2 minutes. Add just enough water to half-cover. Cover the skillet and bring the water to a boil. Reduce the flame to medium-low and simmer for 40 minutes. Then place the green beans on top of the hiziki, cover, and simmer 1–2 minutes. Next, place the sweet corn on top of the green beans and add a small amount of tamari soy sauce for a mild salt taste. Cover and simmer until the green beans and corn become tender but are still brightly colored. Turn up the flame, remove the cover, and cook off all the remaining liquid. Mix the vegetables and place them in a serving dish.

Boiled Kale and Carrots

½ cup carrots, sliced on a
   diagonal
2 cups kale, washed and sliced
water

Yield: Four to five servings.

Place ½ inch of water in a pot and bring it to a boil. Add the carrots and boil 1–2 minutes. Remove the carrots from the pot, drain them, and place them in a bowl. Add the kale. Cover and simmer 1–2 minutes. Remove the kale drain it, and place it in the serving bowl with the carrots. Mix and serve.

Amasake Peach Pudding

1 quart amasake
2 cups peaches, washed and
  sliced
4–6 teaspoons kuzu, diluted in
  4–6 teaspoons of water

Yield: Four to five servings.

Place the amasake and peaches in a saucepan and bring it to a boil. Reduce the flame and simmer until the peaches are soft. Reduce the flame to low and add the diluted kuzu, stirring constantly to prevent lumping. When the mixture thickens, simmer 1–2 minutes. Pour the pudding into a bowl or into individual dessert cups. It may be enjoyed either warm or slightly chilled.

Bancha Tea

1 tablespoon bancha twigs
1 quart water

Yield: Four to five servings.

For a strong beverage, first place the twigs in a dry stainless steel skillet and roast them for several minutes. For a lighter tea, simply place the twigs in a teakettle without roasting. Add the water and place the kettle over a high flame. Bring to a boil, then reduce the flame to low. For a mild tea, simmer 2–3 minutes. You can simmer the twigs for up to 10 minutes if you prefer strong tea. Serve hot.

Chapter Five

NATURAL HOME CARES

Every day, millions of people take tablets and pills for minor complaints such as headaches, stomach upsets, colds, and flu. The root of these common problems is imbalance in the diet, together with changes in the weather and climate. Since medications do not change the underlying causes of these conditions, they tend to return again and again.

In the macrobiotic view, symptoms such as these can be beneficial. Although they may be unpleasant to experience, they help the body to discharge excess and remain free of more serious illness. Minor problems can often be managed at home by changing one's way of eating (especially by avoiding the foods that are producing imbalance), preparing a variety of special dishes, and applying simple forms of home care.

Symptoms such as diarrhea, coughing, sneezing, and fever normally occur when the body discharges excess caused by dietary imbalances such as too much fat, oil, simple sugar, or liquid. In some cases, excess is discharged in the form of skin diseases, including acne and eczema. Acne, for example, is simply the discharge of surplus fat, oil, and sugar through the skin.

To treat acne and other skin conditions, many young people are advised to take daily doses of antibiotics—in some cases, for several years. Using antibiotics in this manner depresses the body's natural immunity and depletes beneficial microorganisms in the intestines. The person's ability to discharge is also diminished. As a result, excess that would normally be discharged is held inside the body. Once trapped, it may accumulate in the breasts, reproductive organs, or lymphatic system. There are alternatives to treating acne with antibiotics. A less symptomatic acne treatment would involve changing the diet and avoiding the types of foods that cause it to develop. Rather than weakening natural immunity, this approach can actually cause the body's immune response to become stronger and more reactive.

Likewise, if a woman with skin problems continues to take in things such as cheese, butter, ice cream, hamburgers, and soft drinks—all of which contain excessive factors—she may ultimately develop cysts or tumors in the breasts or reproductive tract. In men, hard fats often build up in the prostate gland, leading to enlargement. These conditions represent the accumulation of excessive factors which the body is no longer able to discharge. If this process continues unchanged, cancer may be the end result.

More than two thousand years ago, Hippocrates said, "Let thy medicine be thy food, and thy food be thy medicine." This chapter describes a variety of natural preparations that can be made at home in the kitchen. They can help relieve minor ailments such as colds, coughing, skin discharges, fever, and digestive upsets. When properly prepared and administered, these traditional home remedies are completely safe and do not weaken natural immunity. They have been used as a part of preventive lifestyles for thousands of years.

However, the special drinks and other forms of home care listed in this chapter should not be substituted for qualified medical advice when it is necessary. Therefore, persons with serious conditions are advised to contact a physician at their earliest opportunity. In addition, all readers are encouraged to contact a local macrobiotic teacher or macrobiotic center for guidance on the appropriate uses of these natural home cares.

The home cares listed here are best prepared fresh, as needed, and used immediately. Teas should be drunk hot. It is best not to prepare items in this chapter far in advance of use, in large quantities, or to refrigerate, store, or reheat them. For this reason, readers can conclude that all recipes in this chapter will yield one to several servings, depending on the recipe and serving size chosen.

DRINKS AND CONDIMENTS

Azuki Bean Tea

Azuki beans are small and compact in size, oblong in shape, and red or brown in color. They contain less fat and oil than other beans, and in the Far East, where they originated, are considered an "honorary grain." They are enjoyed as a small side dish, in soups, cooked with grains, and in desserts. They have become a staple in many macrobiotic and natural food diets.

Of the varieties of azuki beans available today, higher-grade beans—those with a deep red or maroon color and shiny surface—are preferred for use in home care over those with a dull surface or faded color. High-grade azuki beans are grown in northern Japan in the mineral-rich soil on the island of Hokkaido. They are carefully selected after harvesting so that they are generally uniform in color and shininess. For ordinary daily use, any variety is fine. But for use in health recovery, the higher-grade beans are recommended.

Tea made from high-grade azuki beans can be used to strengthen the kidneys and soften hard stools. The intestines and kidneys are major organs of discharge. It is important that they function properly in order to keep the body free of toxic accumulation. To prepare azuki bean tea, place 1 cup of washed azuki beans in a pot; add 3–4 cups of water and a strip of kombu about an inch long. Bring the water to a boil, cover, reduce the flame to low, and simmer 30–45 minutes. Strain out the liquid. Azuki bean tea can be used for several days or longer. Use it along with other beverages. The leftover beans can be put in soups or cooked with rice.

Bancha Twig Tea

Bancha tea is picked in midsummer from the large and mature leaves, stems, and twigs of the tea bush. The teas that come from these various parts of the plant are called, respectively, bancha leaf tea, bancha stem tea, and bancha twig tea. Traditionally picked by hand in the high mountains, the bancha leaves, stems, and twigs are roasted and cooled up to four separate times in large iron cauldrons. This procedure, as well as the late harvest (at a time when the caffeine has naturally receded from the tea bush), makes for a tea containing virtually no caffeine or tannin. This is especially true of the stem and twig teas.

Unlike other teas, which are acidic, bancha is slightly alkaline and thus has a soothing, beneficial effect on digestion, blood quality, and the mind. It is entirely safe for even infants and small children to drink. In most macrobiotic households, bancha is the most commonly consumed beverage, usually served after every meal and between meals.

Bancha twig tea is sometimes called kukicha tea, from the Japanese words for "twig tea." To prepare it, place a tablespoonful of twigs in a quart of water and bring the water to a boil. Reduce the flame to low and simmer 3–5 minutes (for a mild tea) or 10–15 minutes (for a stronger beverage).

Daikon Tea 1

Daikon, or white radish, is an indispensable part of traditional Far Eastern cuisine and is now grown in America. The smaller, thinner variety, shaped somewhat like a carrot, grows more quickly than the large varieties and has a strong, sharp taste. The big, juicy ones grow up to several feet in length and are sweeter.

Tea made from grated raw daikon has traditionally been used to help reduce fever by inducing sweating. It is not recommended for someone with a weakened condition or for small children. To prepare this tea, grate 1–2 tablespoons of daikon radish, and place it in a teacup. Add $1/4$–$1/2$ teaspoon of fresh grated ginger and a tablespoon of tamari soy sauce. Pour weak hot bancha tea or boiling water over the ingredients. Stir and drink hot. In general, it is best not to use this tea for more than three consecutive days unless you receive an individualized recommendation from a macrobiotic counselor.

Daikon Tea 2

This type of daikon tea can be used to induce urination and calm and relax the body. Grate a small amount of daikon and place it in a piece of cheesecloth. Squeeze 2 tablespoons of juice through the cloth and mix it with about 6 tablespoons of water. Place the liquid in a saucepan and add a pinch of sea salt. Bring to a boil, reduce the flame to low, and simmer for about a minute. Drink this tea hot, and only once per day. It is better not to use this drink for more that three days in a row unless a qualified macrobiotic teacher suggests otherwise.

Daikon Tea 3

This daikon drink helps dissolve deposits of fat and mucus in the body. Place 1 tablespoon of fresh grated daikon in a teacup. Add 1 teaspoon of tamari soy sauce and pour hot bancha tea over the mixture. Drink hot. As with the other daikon teas, it is usually better not to use this drink for more than two or three days unless otherwise indicated.

Daikon-Carrot Drink

Grated daikon and carrot can be used to help the body discharge fats and dissolve hardened accumulations in the intestinal tract. Grate 1 tablespoon each of fresh daikon and carrot. Place 2 cups of water in a saucepan. Add the daikon and carrot and a pinch of sea salt. Bring the water to a boil, reduce the flame to low, and simmer for 5–8 minutes.

Dried Daikon Tea

This drink can be used to help reduce fever in a person who is unable to use raw grated daikon. Place ¼ cup of dried daikon in a saucepan and add 2 cups of water. Bring the water to a boil, reduce the flame to low, and cover the saucepan. Simmer for about 10 minutes. Drink hot.

Grated Daikon Garnish

Grated raw daikon can be used as a garnish that will aid in the digestion of oily or fatty foods such as tempura or mochi. It can also help the body metabolize the oils and fats found in fish and other animal foods. To prepare this garnish, grate 1–2 tablespoons of fresh uncooked daikon and sprinkle several drops of tamari soy sauce over it. You may also add a dab of fresh grated ginger for a slightly stronger garnish. Place several tablespoonfuls on the plate along with your food.

Dandelion Root Tea

Wild dandelion greens have traditionally been eaten in Southern Europe and other temperate areas of the world. They may be prepared as a lightly boiled salad and are usually cooked together with their roots. They may also be sautéed in oil or cooked in a little water. Dandelion greens give strength and vitality, are a good source of fiber, and contribute to smooth digestion. In addition, dandelion root and greens have traditionally been used to strengthen the heart and small intestine and cleanse the liver. Dandelion is especially effective when freshly picked in the early spring.

To prepare dandelion tea, place a quart of water and a tablespoonful of finely chopped dandelion root in a saucepan. Bring to a boil, cover, and reduce the flame to low. Simmer for about 8–10 minutes. Drink one cup hot.

Fresh Lotus Root Tea

In Far Eastern countries, lotus root has been known for centuries as being effective in easing respiratory problems, including coughs and congestion. The root of the lotus flower plant grows underwater in segmented lengths, is light brown in color, and contains hollow chambers. It can be regularly included in the diet in a variety of dishes—with other root vegetables or with sea-vegetables—and can be used in home cares. To prepare lotus root tea, wash and grate a 4-inch piece of lotus root. Wrap it in a piece of cheesecloth and squeeze all of the liquid into a measuring cup.

Add an equal amount of water to the lotus juice and pour the liquid into a saucepan. Add a small pinch of sea salt and bring the water to a boil. Reduce the flame to low and simmer for 3–5 minutes. Drink 1–2 cups of this tea per day for several days. Page 145 has directions for preparing a lotus root plaster for external use.

Gomashio

Gomashio, or "sesame salt," is made from ground roasted sesame seeds and roasted sea salt. It is the most commonly used macrobiotic condiment, and has a salty-bitter taste that balances the natural sweetness of brown rice and other whole grains and vegetables. Gomashio is delicious, and care must be taken not to overconsume it. A half teaspoon to one teaspoon on a bowl of rice is usually plenty.

Gomashio contains high amounts of calcium, iron, and other nutrients, and is an excellent source of polyunsaturated vegetable oil in its whole form. Roasting makes the sesame seeds easier to digest. The combination with roasted salt provides a harmonious balance to the oil. Directions for preparing gomashio are presented on page 55.

The ideal proportion of salt to sesame seeds varies from 1:8 to 1:16 depending on the age and activity level of each person. For active adults, the generally recommended ratio of salt to sesame seeds is slightly higher than for more sedentary adults. For less active adults and for children, the suggested proportion of salt is lower.

Japanese Black Soybean Tea

Black soybeans were used in traditional cultures to strengthen the heart and the female reproductive tract. The sexual organs are a frequent site for the buildup of excess that can lead to a variety of problems, including irregular menstruation, fibroids, and different types of cysts. Problems involving the female reproductive organs are so widespread today that half of all American women have these organs removed by the time they reach the age of sixty. To prepare Japanese black soybean tea, boil 1 cup of washed beans in 3 cups of water for about 30–35 minutes. Strain off the liquid. Drink 1–2 cups of hot tea per day for several days.

Kombu Tea

In traditional medicine, sea-vegetables have been identified especially with strengthening the heart, the blood, and the circulatory system. They are also excellent for the kidneys, the urinary system, and the reproductive organs. They give elasticity to arteries, veins, and organ tissues, contributing to flexibility and the smooth functioning of the body's many interrelated systems. As we saw in Chapter 2, modern scientific research has begun to discover the anti-cancer properties of kombu and other sea-vegetables.

Each type of sea-vegetable, moreover, may have restorative properties as well as preventive ones. Arame, for example, is traditionally used to help relieve female disorders. Hijiki is taken to strengthen the intestines, produce beautiful, shining hair, and purify the blood. Wakame has long been used for cleansing the blood after childbirth. Nori is associated with relieving beriberi and wens. For centuries, Irish moss has been used in Europe to alleviate respiratory ailments. Kombu is taken to reduce high blood pressure and relieve swelling.

Kombu belongs to the *Laminaria* family of sea-vegetables, which includes some types of kelp, carweed, tangle, and other deep-sea varieties. The color of Japanese kombu ranges from dark brown to black and the plant has wide, thick fronds. It is gathered off the southern coast of Hokkaido, Japan's northernmost island. Harvested in middle to late summer by boatmen with long poles, kombu is initially wind- and sun-dried and then stored for two to three years in a dark place before being sold in a variety of grades and sizes.

Like all edible sea-vegetables, kombu is rich in essential minerals and other nutrients. Tea made by boiling kombu supplies valuable nutrients. There are two basic ways to prepare kombu tea:

1. Place 1 quart of water in a pot and add 1 strip of washed kombu, 3–4 inches long. Bring the water to a boil, cover the pot, and simmer until about 2 cups of liquid remain.
2. Place a 6-inch strip of kombu in a 350°F oven and bake for 10–15 minutes or until the kombu is crisp and brittle but not burnt. Then place the roasted kombu in a suribachi and grind it to a fine powder. Place 1/2–1 teaspoon of the powdered kombu in a cup and pour boiling water over it. Stir and drink hot.

You can drink a cup of either of these teas for several days in a row, or can enjoy them as a regular beverage several times per week.

Powdered Lotus Root Tea

Prepackaged powdered lotus root tea is available in most natural and macrobiotic food stores. It can be used when fresh lotus root is not available. Directions for making it are printed on the package. Tea made from powdered lotus root can be used in the same manner as tea made from fresh lotus.

Roasted Barley or Brown Rice Tea

Like bancha, whole grain teas help stabilize the body's overall use of energy. They also help with the gradual elimination of excess factors that have accumulated in the body as a result of the overconsumption of animal fats and proteins. These teas are especially helpful in relieving dry skin (especially on the hands and feet). Brown rice tea may aid in strengthening the lungs and large intestine, and barley tea may fortify the liver and gallbladder. To prepare the tea, place 1–2 tablespoons of roasted barley or ¼ cup of dry-roasted brown rice in a quart of water. Bring to a boil, reduce the flame to low, and simmer for about 10 minutes. Either of these teas can be used daily as one of your staple beverages.

Shiitake Mushroom Tea

Shiitake mushrooms, an ingredient traditionally used in soup stock, have been found to have cancer-inhibiting effects. In 1970, Japanese cancer researchers reported that shiitake markedly inhibited the growth of certain tumors in animals, resulting in "almost complete regression . . . with no sign of toxicity."

Shiitake are originally native to the Far East, and are now grown in America. They are very delicious and, fresh or dried, have been used for centuries to counterbalance heavy animal food intake and for other medicinal purposes. Shiitake tea can be used to relax the overly tight condition that may result from the consumption of too much salt or animal food. To prepare the tea, take 1 shiitake and place it in a saucepan. Add 2 cups of water, bring to a boil, reduce the flame to low, and cover. Simmer, together with a small pinch of sea salt or 1 teaspoon of tamari soy sauce, until 1 cup of water remains. Strain the tea and drink ½ cup at a time while it is still hot.

Tamari-Bancha Tea

Tamari-bancha is easy to make. It promotes circulation and helps neutralize an overly acidic blood condition. It can also help restore vitality and alleviate headaches caused by overconsumption of sugar, alcohol, or other acid-producing foods and beverages. To prepare the tea, pour 1–2 teaspoons of tamari soy sauce into a teacup. Pour hot bancha tea over it and stir. Drink hot.

Tamari-Kuzu Tea

Kuzu is known as "kudzu" in the southern United States, where it is found in abundance. This deep-rooted vine also grows wild in the mountains of Japan, where it is traditionally harvested and processed by hand into a white chalklike substance. Kuzu is often used in macrobiotic cooking as a thickener in sauces, stews, and desserts. Its medicinal properties include strengthening the digestive organs. Tamari-kuzu can be used to fortify digestion, increase vitality, and relieve fatigue.

To prepare it, place a heaping teaspoon of kuzu powder in a saucepan and add 2 teaspoons of water. Mix until the kuzu is completely dissolved. Add a cup of water and continue mixing. Bring the mixture to a boil, reduce the flame to low, and simmer until the kuzu is translucent and thick. Stir constantly to prevent lumping. Add 1/2–1 teaspoon of tamari soy sauce and mix. Simmer the tamari-kuzu for another minute before pouring it into a bowl or cup. Drink it hot.

Umeboshi Tea

Umeboshi plums grow in the warmer southern and middle regions of Japan and are related to the apricot. Traditionally fermented with sea salt and pickled with shiso leaves (which give them a deep reddish-purple color), umeboshi have a tangy flavor, combining sour and salty tastes. They are a very balanced food, give a strong centering energy, and have a wide range of uses in macrobiotic cooking and home care. The sourness of the plums and their strong alkalizing (anti-acid) effects help to strengthen the stomach and digestive organs. Umeboshi can be used to help offset diarrhea, upset stomach, and other digestive disorders, and to neutralize an overacid blood condition.

There are a number of ways to use umeboshi in home cares. To prepare umeboshi tea, take a plum and bake it in the oven until it becomes completely black and crisp. Grind the baked plum in a suribachi until you obtain a fine powder. Place a tablespoonful of the powder in a cup and pour hot water over it. Mix well and drink hot.

Ume-Sho-Bancha Tea

Ume-sho-bancha (umeboshi plus tamari plus bancha) helps fortify the blood and stimulate active circulation. It can be used to help relieve fatigue or weakness and ease a headache, especially when the pain is centered in the front of the head. To prepare, place 1/2–1 plum in a cup with 1/2–1 teaspoon of tamari soy sauce. Add hot bancha tea, stir, and drink hot.

Ume-Sho-Bancha Tea with Ginger

Adding a pinch of grated ginger to ume-sho-bancha makes blood circulation even more active and helps warm the body. Prepare as indicated above, but add ¼ teaspoon of freshly grated ginger. Mix well and drink hot.

Ume-Sho-Kuzu Tea

This preparation combines the effects of umeboshi and kuzu. It can be used to strengthen the intestines and digestive system as a whole and also to restore active energy. In addition, ume-sho-kuzu is frequently used to relieve diarrhea or constipation caused by overly weak or expanded intestines.

In a saucepan, dilute a heaping teaspoonful of kuzu powder in 2 teaspoons of water. Add another cup of water and mix well. Then, remove the pit of an umeboshi plum and add the plum. Bring the water to a boil, stirring constantly to prevent lumping. Reduce the flame to low and simmer until the mixture becomes thick and translucent. When it is nearly ready, add ½–1 teaspoon of tamari soy sauce and simmer for several more seconds. For a lighter preparation, you can also add a small amount of grated ginger at the end. Pour the ume-sho-kuzu into a bowl or cup and drink it hot.

In traditional medicine, gomashio has been used to restore elasticity to the heart and circulatory system. Eating a naturally balanced diet and including foods such as gomashio and sea-vegetables is a safe and effective way of restoring health to this vital system, in contrast to approaches that run the risk of side effects.

Recently, however, rather than changing their diets, many people have begun taking daily doses of aspirin to lower their risk of heart attack and stroke. Aspirin is an extremely yin or expansive product, and it produces a wide range of side effects. Aspirin interferes with the more yang capacity of the blood to clot, and therefore makes it harder for wounds to heal. It can also cause the blood vessels to expand and erupt, resulting in bleeding. Aspirin-induced bleeding occurs more readily in the stomach, intestines, and other organs with a hollow and expanded shape than in those with compact structures like the heart and liver.

Some cardiovascular disorders result from overconsumption of extreme yang foods, such as meat, eggs, cheese, and others that contain plenty of saturated fat and cholesterol. Other cardiovascular problems have an opposite dietary cause. They arise from an overintake of sugar, coffee, soft drinks, milk, ice cream, tropical fruits, and other extreme yin items. Strokes involving ruptures of blood vessels in the brain can be examples of this type of disorder. Researchers have discovered that aspirin doesn't help these conditions; it could, in fact, make them worse.

General dietary change in the direction of macrobiotics is a far safer method to prevent circulatory disorders without the risk of side effects.

COMPRESSES, BODY SCRUBS, AND PLASTERS

Hot Water Body Scrub

A daily body scrub with a hot towel is a simple and effective way to promote overall health and vitality. It stimulates circulation, releases stagnation, and helps break down fats deposited under the skin.

After many years of consuming cheese, chicken, meat, eggs, and other animal foods, many people develop a layer of hard fat just below the skin. This condition occurs in thin people as well as in the overweight, and produces hard, dry skin and a reduced capacity to perspire.

The skin is one of the body's major organs of discharge. When the pores and sweat glands become constricted and blocked with fatty deposits, toxic factors that are normally discharged can start to accumulate. This can lead to the buildup of toxins throughout the body, creating a medium for the eventual development of cancer. It is therefore important to avoid the foods that cause these fats to develop and to practice daily body scrubbing in order to open the pores and allow excess to come out.

Body scrubbing can be done before or after a bath or shower. All you need is a sink with hot water and a medium-sized cotton towel. Turn the hot water on. Hold your towel at either end and run the center part under the stream of hot water. Wring the towel out, and, while it is still hot and steamy, begin to scrub yourself with it. Begin with your hands and fingers and work your way up your arms to the shoulders, neck, and face. Then scrub downward to the chest, upper back, abdomen, lower back, buttocks, legs, feet, and toes. Make sure to scrub your entire body so that the skin turns slightly red and/or until each part becomes warm. You can reheat the towel by running it under the hot water after scrubbing each section or as soon as it starts to cool.

A hot towel body scrub is ideal once or twice a day. When you do it in the morning, it has the effect of vitalizing and energizing you for the day's activity. When you do it in the evening, it releases stress and tension and relaxes and refreshes you. The total body scrub takes only about ten minutes to do.

Hot Towel Compresses

Hot towels can also be used to promote circulation, relax specific areas of the body, and relieve aches and pains. Prepare a hot towel (as for the body scrub described above), fold it into sections, and apply it to the area you wish to treat. Hold it in place until it cools, and then reheat the towel and apply it again. Continue applying the hot towel for 5–10 minutes or until the area becomes red and/or warm.

Ginger Compress

Ginger compresses work like hot towel compresses to stimulate circulation, dissolve stagnation, and relax specific areas of the body. Adding freshly grated ginger to hot water makes the heat even more stimulating and penetrating.

Ginger compresses can be applied alone if you are able to reach the area you wish to treat, or with a partner if the area is hard to reach. To make the compress, you will need a medium-sized piece of fresh ginger root (available at most natural food or Oriental markets), a flat metal grater, some cheesecloth, 3 medium-sized cotton towels, and a medium-to-large pot with a lid.

Grate the ginger root and place a clump about the size of a golf ball in a double layer of cheesecloth. Tie the cheesecloth at the top to form a sack. Then put a gallon of water in a pot and bring it up to, but not over, the boiling point. Just before the water starts to boil, turn the flame down to low.

Hold the cheesecloth sack over the pot and squeeze as much of the ginger juice as you can into the water. Then drop the sack into the pot. Make sure the water doesn't boil, because boiling weakens the effect of the compress. Place the lid on the pot and let the ginger sack simmer in the water for about 5 minutes.

Fold one of the towels lengthwise several times so that it becomes long and thin. Hold it at both ends and dip the middle portion into the hot ginger water. Wring the towel out tightly, and if it is too hot to place on your skin, shake it slightly. Then place the hot towel on the area you wish to treat, and cover it with one of the dry towels to reduce heat loss. With the hot towel still in place, prepare another ginger towel in the same manner. Apply it as soon as the first towel cools, and repeat the procedure, alternating hot towels, every 2–3 minutes until the skin becomes red and/or warm.

The ginger compress is fine for use by normally healthy adults as a part of general health improvement. However, it should not be applied in cases of fever or inflammation. Also, it is recommended that persons with cancer or other serious illnesses use a milder application, such as a simple hot towel compress, unless advised to do otherwise by a qualified macrobiotic teacher.

Ginger Body Scrub

A special body scrub can be done with hot ginger water. Dip a medium-sized cotton towel in the pot of hot ginger water as described for the ginger compress (see above), but instead of applying it to only one area, use it to scrub your entire body. This can be done after the application of a ginger compress or by itself. Many people find plain hot water body scrubbing convenient during the week, and use the ginger body scrub on the weekends when more time is available. One pot of ginger water can be used for two days of body scrubs. Simply reheat the water before using it (don't bring it to a boil).

Mustard Plaster

The old-fashioned mustard plaster stimulates blood and body fluid circulation and loosens stagnation, especially in the case of chest colds or congestion. To prepare it, add 1 cup hot water to 1 cup dry powdered mustard and mix well. The consistency should be thick, not soupy. Spread the mixture onto a paper towel and sandwich it between two thick cotton bath towels. Apply this "sandwich" to the skin and leave it on until the skin becomes warm and/or red. Then remove it, and wipe the skin with a damp towel to remove any mustard liquid.

It is a good idea to have another person apply the plaster for you, as heat from the mustard can make you drowsy. When giving children a mustard plaster, mix 1/2 cup mustard powder, 1/2 cup whole wheat pastry flour, and 1 cup water, and apply the plaster for a shorter period of time, and only until the skin becomes slightly warm or pink. If the skin starts to burn or itch at any time during the application, take the plaster off.

Tofu Plaster

Raw tofu is milder yet more effective than ice in drawing out a fever. To prepare a tofu plaster, squeeze the water from a 1-pound block of tofu and mash the tofu in a suribachi with 1/4–1/3 cup whole wheat pastry flour and 1 level teaspoon freshly grated ginger. Mix all of the ingredients thoroughly and spread the mixture in a layer about 1/2 inch thick on a clean piece of cotton cheesecloth or a cotton towel. Apply the plaster directly—tofu side to the skin—to the forehead, back of the head, or other exposed part of the body. Change it every couple of hours, or leave it on until the tofu becomes warm or the fever drops.

Green Vegetable Plaster

Raw green vegetables can also be used to lower fevers if tofu is not available. To prepare vegetable plasters, chop a bunch of washed greens (such as collard, kale, or watercress) very finely. Place them in a suribachi and grind them thoroughly. If the greens are very watery, mix in a littly pastry flour to hold the mixture together. Place the mashed greens on a piece of cotton cheesecloth or cotton linen to form a layer about ½ inch thick. Apply the plaster directly to the forehead or another exposed part of the body. The vegetable mixture should come directly in contact with the skin. Change the plaster every several hours, or leave it on until the greens become warm.

Tofu-Green Vegetable Plaster

This plaster combines the effects of raw tofu and greens and can also be used to bring down a fever. To prepare it, chop ⅓ cup of leafy greens very finely and mash them in a suribachi. Place 1 pound tofu and 1 level teaspoon grated ginger in the suribachi and grind the ingredients to obtain a thick paste. Place the paste on a clean piece of cotton cheesecloth or towel creating a layer about ½ inch thick. Apply as described for the green vegetable plaster (see above).

Salt Pack

Roasted salt can be used to warm and soothe any part of the body—for example, the shoulders, when aches and pains are felt there. It can also be applied to the abdomen to help relieve diarrhea or to ease menstrual cramps.

To prepare a salt pack, dry-roast salt in a stainless steel skillet. Stir it from time to time until it becomes very hot. Place the hot salt in a thick cotton sack or pillowcase. Don't use a sack made of synthetic material, as the hot salt will cause it to melt. Tie the sack with a piece of string and then wrap it in a thick cotton bath towel. Place it on the area you wish to treat, and leave it on until it cools. Once it cools, you may replace it with another salt pack if you wish, but one application is usually enough. Save the salt, as it can be re-roasted several more times. Discard it once it turns grey, however, as it will no longer retain heat at this point.

Lotus Root Plaster

Freshly-grated lotus root can be used to draw stagnated mucus from the sinuses, nose, throat, and bronchi. Wash a piece of lotus root and grate it on a flat metal grater. Mix the grated lotus with 10–15 percent whole wheat pastry flour and 5 percent freshly grated ginger. Thus, 80–85 percent of the mixture will consist of grated lotus root. (You can obtain the right proportions by using 16–17 times more grated lotus than flour, and about twice as much flour as ginger.) Spread a half-inch layer of this mixture on a piece of cotton linen and apply the plaster so that the mixture comes into direct contact with the skin. Leave it on for several hours or overnight. This plaster can be used daily for up to ten days, or until stagnated deposits of mucus begin to be discharged. A hot ginger or hot water compress may be applied to the skin before the lotus plaster is put on to warm the area and loosen stagnation.

Dark Sesame Oil

Sesame oil can be used to keep the skin healthy and smooth. It is helpful in relieving minor burns or chapped skin. For burns, first soak the area in cool salt water, then apply a piece of tofu until the pain is gone. Then gently rub dark sesame oil on the area. For chapped skin, gently rub the oil on the affected area as needed.

BATHS AND SOAKS

Daikon Hip Bath

Reproductive disorders have become epidemic in modern society. According to present estimates, one in every five American couples is infertile. An estimated 40 percent of women have Premenstrual Syndrome (PMS), including 3 percent with severe cases. In addition, 40 percent of women have fibroid tumors. Surgeons annually perform over 4 million operations on female genital organs—including about 700,000 hysterectomies. One baby out of every five born today is delivered by Cesarean section.

The reproductive organs are a frequent site for the accumulation of excess. In women, these accumulations may not only take the form of fibroid tumors and dermoid cysts, but also, in extreme cases, cancer of the ovaries, uterus, or cervix. Vaginal discharge, a common condition today, is an indication that excess is beginning to build up in this part of the body.

In men, the prostate gland is often affected by the buildup of excess. The first signs of accumulation are often small microscopic nodules, known as prostatic concretions, that appear in the fluid secreted by the gland. If plenty of hard fats are consumed—especially those in cheese, butter, meat, and eggs—and iced or chilled foods and beverages are taken often, the concretions may harden and calcify in a manner similiar to kidney stones. Prostatic concretions may accumulate in the gland itself in the form of cysts.

In traditional macrobiotic medicine, the daikon hip bath is frequently used by women to relieve reproductive disorders. Ideally, the bathwater should contain dried daikon leaves (turnip greens or arame sea-vegetable can be used when daikon greens are not available). To dry daikon greens, simply hang up bunches of fresh leaves and leave them until they turn brown and brittle. To prepare the bath, place 4–5 bunches of dried leaves or a double handful of arame in a large pot. Add about 4–5 quarts of water and bring to a boil. Reduce the flame to medium and boil until the water turns brown. Add a handful of sea salt and stir well to dissolve.

Then, run hot water in the bathtub and add the dried daikon mixture together with another large handful of sea salt. Use only enough water to cover the body from the waist down. Sit in the tub and cover your upper body with a thick cotton towel to prevent chills and absorb perspiration. If the bath water begins to cool, add more hot water and stay in the bath for ten to twelve minutes.

The hot bath will cause the circulation to increase in your lower body; your skin may turn very red. This circulation will loosen fat and mucus deposits in the pelvic region.

Following the hip bath, douche with a special solution. Prepare this either by squeezing the juice from half a lemon into warm bancha tea or by adding one to two teaspoons of brown rice vinegar to warm bancha tea. Add a three-finger pinch of sea salt, stir, and use as a douche. The douching solution helps dislodge deposits of mucus and fat that have been loosened during the bath. The hip bath and douche can be repeated every day for up to ten days. During this time, it is important to eat well and to avoid foods that contribute to the buildup of excess in the reproductive tract.

Daikon Leaf Skin Wash

Dried daikon (or turnip) greens are also helpful in relieving skin conditions such as eczema, acne, and impetigo, among others. Prepare the dried leaves as indicated for the daikon hip bath (above). However, rather than pouring the mixture into the bathtub, dip a cotton towel into the pot and squeeze it lightly. Apply it to the affected area, making repeated applications until the skin turns red or begins to tingle.

Rice Bran (Nuka) Skin Wash or Bath

Nuka, or rice bran, can be purchased at most natural food stores. It has been used for centuries to promote healthy skin and to improve skin disorders. To prepare a skin wash, wrap the nuka in cheesecloth and tie it to create a sack. Place the cheesecloth sack in warm water, squeeze, and shake. The nuka will dissolve, the water will turn yellowish, and a white foam may form on the surface. Lightly wash the affected area several times with a towel or facecloth that has been dipped in the nuka water.

A person with skin problems can also take a bath in which nuka has been dissolved. Put about 3 to 5 tablespoons of nuka into a white cotton sock or a sack made of thin cotton cloth or cheesecloth. Tie the sock (or sack) so that the nuka does not fall out. Place it in the bathwater and squeeze it until a milky liquid comes out. Mix the milky liquid in with the bathwater and use it to wash the skin, especially including the areas affected by the disorder. Rice bran contains a natural oil that helps the skin return to a smooth and healthy condition. You can also wash your hair in the nuka water.

If you cannot find rice bran, you can substitute about 1/4 cup of rolled oats instead. Nuka or oat applications may also be used to ease the itching and discomfort of poison ivy or insect bites.

Ginger Water Foot Soak

Often, years of consuming animal proteins and fats cause hard calluses to build up on the bottoms of the feet and toes. These deposits interfere with the smooth exchange of energy between the feet and the environment, especially the flow of energy that runs through the organ meridians that connect to the toes. Soaking the feet in a shallow basin filled with hot ginger water helps to soften these deposits and increases overall circulation. The foot soak can be done immediately after a ginger compress or body scrub. Simply pour the hot ginger water into a basin. Place both feet in the basin and let them soak for five to ten minutes. Then rub them briskly with a dry cotton towel.

ONE STEP FURTHER

Today, it is becoming apparent that the degenerative diseases of the twentieth century—cancer and heart disease in particular—are the result of our modern lifestyle. They are caused not by germs or microbes, but by everyday patterns of living, especially our choice of foods.

Staying healthy has now become the responsibility of each of us as individuals. The choices we make today, from the foods we place on our dinner tables, to the types of exercise we pursue, all influence our health tomorrow.

With accumulating evidence linking diet with cancer and other degenerative diseases, the question now is not *why* we should change our diets, but *why not*. For the past quarter century, macrobiotic education has offered a sensible approach to reducing the risk of cancer through better diet and a more natural way of life. The essential principles of macrobiotics—such as reducing the intake of fat, sugar, and refined and processed foods, and basing the diet around whole grains, beans, and fresh vegetables—are now supported by sound nutritional research. The art of macrobiotic cooking, practiced in thousands of homes around the world, offers a time-tested method for applying preventive dietary guidelines in the kitchen. A cancer prevention lifestyle can begin with your next meal. It is our hope that both the dietary and way-of-life guidelines, menus and recipes, and basic home cares presented in this book will help guide you toward a healthier and brighter future, free from cancer and chronic illness.

Glossary

Agar-agar.   A white gelatin derived from a sea-vegetable, used in making aspics.

Amazake.   A sweetener or refreshing drink made from sweet rice and koji starter that is allowed to ferment into a thick liquid. Hot amazake is a delicious sweet beverage. It may be referred to as amazake or amasake.

Arrowroot.   A starch flour processed from the root of an American native plant. It is used as a thickening agent, similar to cornstarch or *kuzu*, for making sauces, stews, gravies, and desserts.

Azuki Bean.   A small, dark red bean imported from Japan, but also grown in the United States. Good when cooked with *kombu** sea-vegetable. This bean may also be referred to as aduki or adzuki.

Bancha Tea.   Correctly named kukicha, bancha tea is made by steeping the stems and leaves from mature Japanese tea bushes. This tea aids in digestion and contains no chemical dyes. Bancha makes an excellent breakfast or after-dinner beverage.

Barley, Pearl.   A particular strain of barley native to China, pearl barley grows easily in colder climates. It is good in stews and mixed with other grains such as rice. It is effective in breaking down animal fats in the body.

Black Sesame Seeds.   Small black seeds, occasionally used as a garnish or in black *gomashio*, a condiment. A different variety of seed from the common tan sesame seed.

Brown Rice.   Whole, unpolished rice. It is available in three varieties: short, medium, and long-grain, and contains an ideal balance of minerals, protein, and carbohydrates.

Burdock.   A hardy plant that grows wild throughout the U.S. The long, dark burdock root is delicious in soups, stews, and sea-vegetable dishes,

---

*Italicized words are defined in glossary.

or sautéed with carrots. It is highly valued in macrobiotic cooking for its strengthening qualities.

Chemical Additives. Any of the various artificial flavorings, coloring agents, or preservatives, not naturally found in foods, that are used in refining and processing. Over three thousand chemical additives have been approved by the U.S. Food and Drug Administration.

Chinese Cabbage. A large, leafy vegetable with pale green tops and thick white stems. Sometimes called nappa, this juicy, slightly sweet vegetable is good in soups and stews, vegetable dishes, and pickled.

Cholesterol. A compound manufactured in the human body, important in the structure of membranes and the formation of certain hormones. Cholesterol is also a constituent of all animal products. Medical studies point to a relationship between excess consumption of cholesterol and the incidence of cancer.

Complex Carbohydrates. Those starches, known chemically as polysaccharides, that provide the body with a high proportion of usable energy over a period of several hours. Complex carbohydrates are the major components of the macrobiotic diet. A source of energy, they are supplied primarily by whole grains, vegetables, and beans.

Daikon. A long, white radish. Besides making a delicious side dish, daikon is a specific aid in dissolving fat and *mucus* deposits that have accumulated as a result of past animal food intake. Grated daikon aids in the digestion of oily foods.

Dried Daikon. Many natural food stores now carry packaged daikon that has been shredded and dried. This is especially good cooked with *kombu* and seasoned with a little *tamari*. Soaking dried daikon before use brings out its natural sweetness.

Dried Tofu. Tofu that has been naturally dehydrated by freezing. Used in soups, stews, vegetable, and sea-vegetable dishes. Less fatty than regular tofu. See *Tofu*.

Dulse. A reddish-purple sea-vegetable used in soups, salads, and vegetable dishes. Very high in protein, Vitamin A, iodine, and phosphorous. Used for centuries in European cooking, dulse is now harvested on both sides of the North Atlantic (including off the coasts of Maine and Massachusetts).

Fiber. The indigestible portion of whole foods; particularly, the bran of whole grains and the outer skin of legumes, vegetables, and fruits. Fiber facilitates the passage of waste through the intestines. Foods that are refined, processed, or peeled are low in fiber. Medical studies point to a positive relationship between fiber consumption and low incidence of cancer of the colon.

Fu. A dried wheat *gluten* product. Available in thin sheets or thick round cakes. Used in soups, stews, and vegetable dishes. High in protein.

Ginger. A spicy, pungent, golden-colored root, used as a garnish or seasoning in cooking. Also used in such remedies as the ginger compress.

Gluten (Wheat). The sticky substance that remains after the bran has been kneaded and rinsed from whole wheat flour. Used to make *seitan* and *fu*.

Gomashio. A condiment made from roasted, ground sesame seeds and *sea salt*. Gomashio is a rich source of minerals and whole oil and can be sprinkled lightly on rice and other grains.

Goma Dulse Powder. A condiment made from ground, baked *dulse* and sesame seeds. Also rich in minerals and other essential nutrients. Used on hot cereals.

Green Nori Flakes. A sea-vegetable condiment made from a certain type of *nori*, different from the packaged variety. The flakes are rich in iron, calcium, and Vitamin A. Can be sprinkled on whole grains, vegetables, salads, and other dishes.

Hiziki. A dark brown sea-vegetable that turns black when dried. It has a wiry consistency, may be strong-tasting, and is high in calcium and protein. Hiziki imported from Japan or havested off the coast of Maine is available dried and packaged in most natural food stores.

Hokkaido Pumpkin. There are two varieties of Hokkaido pumpkin. One has a deep orange color and the other has a light green skin similar to Hubbard squash. Hokkaido pumpkins are available at many natural food stores and by mail order. They have a tough outer skin and are very sweet inside.

Japanese Black Soybeans. A special type of soybean grown in Japan. It may be used medicinally to treat female reproductive problems. In cooking, black beans are used in soups and side dishes.

Kinpira. A sautéed *burdock* or burdock-and-carrot dish that is seasoned with *tamari*. This hearty root vegetable dish imparts strength and vitality.

Kombu. A wide, thick, dark green sea-vegetable that grows in deep ocean water. Often cooked with vegetables and beans; and used in making condiments, candy, and soup stocks. A single strip of kombu may be re-used several times to flavor soups. Kombu is rich in essential minerals. Medical studies have reported kombu's effectiveness in helping to prevent a variety of cancers.

Kuzu. A white starch made from the root of the wild kuzu plant. In the U.S., the plant is often called kudzu. Used in making soups, sauces, gravies, desserts, and for medicinal purposes.

Lotus Root. The root and seeds of a water lily which is brown-skinned with a hollow, chambered, off-white inside. Especially good for the respiratory organs. The seeds are used in grain, bean, and sea-vegetable dishes.

Macrobiotics. An approach to balanced living, based on a balanced diet, moderate exercise, harmony with the environment, and an understanding of the philosophic principles of *yin* and *yang*. George Ohsawa was the first to recognize how these traditional concepts could be applied to modern living.

Millet.   This small, yellow grain, which comes in many varieties, can be eaten on a regular basis. It can be used in soups or vegetable dishes, or eaten as a cereal.

Mirin.   A wine made from whole grain sweet rice. Used occasionally as a seasoning in vegetable or sea-vegetable dishes.

Miso.   A fermented grain or bean paste made from ingredients such as soybeans, barley, and rice. There are many varieties of miso now available. Barley (mugi) or soybean (hatcho) miso is usually recommended for daily use. Miso is especially good for the the circulatory and digestive organs. It is high in protein and Vitamin B_{12}.

Miso, Puréed.   Miso that has been reduced to a texture that will allow it to blend easily with other ingredients. To purée miso, place it in a bowl or *suribachi* and add enough water or broth to make a smooth paste. Blend with a wooden pestle or spoon.

Mochi.   A rice cake or dumpling made from cooked, pounded sweet rice.

Mucus.   Secretion of mucous membranes, normally serving to protect and lubricate main parts of the body. Illness, environmental pollution, smoking, and the consumption of excess fats, sugar, and flour products can stimulate the overproduction of *mucus* and clog body passageways, preventing the body from expelling harmful substances.

Nishime.   A method of cooking in which different combinations of vegetables, sea-vegetables, or soybean products are cut in large pieces and simmered for a long time over a low flame. Nishime is seasoned with *tamari* or *miso*, and cooked until almost all the water in the pot is gone. The ingredients become soft, sweet, and easily digested. Also referred to as waterless cooking.

Nori.   Thin sheets of dried sea-vegetable that are black or dark purple when dried. Nori is often roasted over a flame until green. It is used as a garnish, wrapped around *rice balls* in making *sushi*, or cooked with *tamari* as a condiment.   Rich in Vitamin A and protein, nori also contains calcium, iron, Vitamins B_1, B_2, C, and D.

Ohitashi.   A method of boiling for leafy green vegetables sliced or whole. Water is boiled, vegetables are added and boiled from several seconds to a minute. Sometimes referred to as blanching.

Organic Foods.   Foods grown and harvested without the use of synthetically-compounded chemical fertilizers, pesticides, herbicides, and fungicides.

Polyunsaturated Fats.   Term used to describe the molecular structure of the fats that are present in vegetable oils and other whole foods, including fish. While polyunsaturates are more healthful than saturated fats, overconsumption may lead to elevated fatty acid (triglyceride) levels in the bloodstream.

Pressed Salad. Very thinly sliced or shredded fresh vegetables, combined with a pickling agent such as *sea salt, umeboshi*, grain vinegar, or *tamari*, and placed in a special pickle press. In the pickling process, many of the enzymes and vitamins are retained while the vegetables become easier to digest.

Preventive Diet. A diet whose goal is to reduce the risks of contracting a disease. Preventive diets exclude foods that have been linked to the formation of a disease and include foods that have been linked to the prevention of that disease.

Rice Balls. Rice shaped into balls or triangles, usually with a piece of *umeboshi* in the center, and wrapped in toasted *nori* or *shiso* leaves to completely cover. Pickles, seeds, vegetables, fried *tofu*, and other ingredients can be placed in the center to create a variety of tastes. Rice balls can also be coated with whole or ground sesame seeds.

Saturated Fats. Term used to describe the molecular structure of most of the fats found in red meats, dairy products, and other animal foods. Medical studies have linked the overconsumption of animal fats to the incidence of cancer.

Sea Salt. Salt obtained from evaporated sea water, as opposed to rock salt. It is either sun-baked or kiln-baked. High in trace minerals, it contains no harmful chemicals, sugar, or iodine.

Seitan. Wheat gluten cooked in *tamari, kombu*, and water. Seitan can be made at home or purchased ready-made at many natural food stores. Many people use it as a meat substitute.

Sesame Butter. A nut butter obtained by roasting and grinding sesame seeds until smooth and creamy. Used like peanut butter or in salad dressings and sauces.

Shiitake Mushrooms. Dried shiitake are imported from Japan. Fresh shiitake, grown in the U.S., have recently come on the market. Either type can be used in soup stocks or vegetable dishes, and dried shiitake are used in medicinal preparations. These mushrooms are effective in helping the body to discharge excess salt and animal fats.

Shio Kombu. Pieces of *kombu* cooked for a long time in *tamari* and used as a condiment. Use only a few pieces at a time, as shio kombu has a strong, salty taste.

Shio Nori. Pieces of *nori* cooked for a long time in *tamari* and water. Used occasionally as a condiment, shio nori is particularly tasty as a relish.

Shiso. A red, pickled leaf. The plant is known in English as the beefsteak plant. It is used to color *umeboshi* plums and as a condiment. Sometimes called chiso.

Simple Sugars. A source of quick, but short-lasting, energy. Simple sugars include sucrose (table sugar), fructose, glucose (dextrose), and lactose (milk sugar). Up to fifty percent of the carbohydrates consumed in the average modern diet are simple sugars.

Suribachi. A special, serrated, glazed clay bowl. Used with a pestle, called a *surikogi*, for grinding and puréeing foods. An essential item in a macrobiotic kitchen, the suribachi can be used in a variety of ways to make condiments, spreads, dressings, baby foods, nut butters, and medicinal preparations.

Surikogi. A wooden pestle that is used with a *suribachi*. Used to make *gomashio*, sea-vegetable powders, and other condiments, and to mash foods to obtain a creamy consistency.

Sushi. Rice rolled with vegetables, fish, or pickles, wrapped in *nori*, and sliced in rounds. Sushi is becoming increasingly popular throughout the U.S. The best-quality macrobiotic sushi is made with brown rice and other natural ingredients.

Sushi Mat. Very thin strips of bamboo that are fastened together with cotton thread so that they can be rolled tightly yet allow air to pass through freely. Used in rolling sushi, and also to cover freshly-cooked foods or leftovers.

Sweet Brown Rice. A sweeter-tasting, more glutinous variety of rice. Used in *mochi*, ohagi, dumplings, and other dishes, it is often used in cooking for festive occasions.

Tamari. Name given by George Ohsawa to traditional, naturally made soy sauce to distinguish it from commercial, chemically processed varieties. Original tamari is the liquid poured off during the process of making hatcho *miso*. The best quality tamari soy sauce is naturally fermented over two summers and is made from round soybeans and *sea salt* that is not highly refined.

Taro. A type of potato with a thick, dark brown, hairy skin. Used as a vegetable or in the preparation of plasters for medicinal purposes. Also called albi.

Tekka. A condiment made from hatcho *miso*, sesame oil, *burdock*, *lotus root*, carrot, and *ginger* root, sautéed on a low flame for several hours.

Tempeh. A dish made from split soybeans, water, and a special bacteria, that is allowed to ferment for several hours. Tempeh is eaten in Indonesia and Sri Lanka as a staple food. It is available prepacked, ready to prepare, in some natural food stores. Rich in Vitamin B_{12} and protein.

Tofu. Soybean curd, made from soybeans and nigari (a coagulant taken from salt water). Used in soups, vegetable dishes, dressings, etc., tofu is high in protein and does not contain animal fats. See *Dried Tofu*.

Udon. Japanese noodles made from wheat, whole wheat, or whole wheat and unbleached white flour. Udon generally have a lighter flavor than soba (buckwheat) noodles.

Umeboshi. Salty, pickled plums. Umeboshi plums stimulate the appetite and digestion and aid in maintaining an alkaline blood quality. *Shiso* leaves are usually added to the plums during pickling to impart a reddish color and natural flavoring.

Umeboshio Vinegar.   A salty, sour vinegar made from umeboshi plums. Diluted with water and used in sweet and sour sauces, salads, salad dressings, etc.

Unsaturated Fats.   See *Polyunsaturated Fats*.

Wakame.   A long, thin, green sea-vegetable used in making soups, salads, and vegetable dishes. High in protein, iron, and magnesium, wakame has a sweet taste and delicate texture and is especially good in *miso* soup.

Wheat Berries.   The grains of whole wheat are often called wheat berries. Wheat berries are good when soaked and pressure-cooked together with brown rice.

Wild Rice.   A wild grass that grows in water and is harvested by hand. Eaten traditionally by native Americans in Minnesota and other areas.

Yang.   In macrobiotics, energy or movement that has a centripetal or inward direction. One of the two antagonistic, yet complementary, forces that together describe all phenomena, yang is traditionally symbolized by a triangle ($\triangle$).

Yin.   In macrobiotics, energy or movement that has a centrifugal or outward direction and results in expansion. One of the two antagonistic, yet complementary, forces that together describe all phenomena, yin is traditionally symbolized by an inverted triangle ($\triangledown$).

Resources

MACROBIOTIC WAY OF LIFE SEMINAR

The Macrobiotic Way of Life Seminar is an introductory program offered by the Kushi Institute in Boston. It includes classes in macrobiotic cooking, home care, kitchen setup, lectures on the philosophy of macrobiotics and the standard diet, and individual way of life guidance. It is presented monthly and includes introductory and intermediate level programs. Information on the Way of Life Seminar is available from:

The Kushi Institute
17 Station Street
Brookline, Massachusetts 02146
(617) 738-0045

MACROBIOTIC RESIDENTIAL SEMINAR

The Macrobiotic Residential Seminar is an introductory program offered at the Kushi Foundation Berkshires Center in Becket, Massachusetts. It is a one week live-in program that includes hands-on training in macrobiotic cooking and home care, lectures on the philosophy and practice of macrobiotics, and meals prepared by a specially trained cooking staff. It is presented monthly and includes introductory and intermediate levels. Information on the Macrobiotic Residential Seminar is available from:

Kushi Foundation Berkshires Center
Box 7
Becket, Massachusetts 01223
(413) 623-5742

KUSHI INSTITUTE LEADERSHIP STUDIES

For those who wish to study further, the Kushi Institute offers instruction for individuals who wish to become trained and certified macrobiotic teachers. Leadership training programs are also offered at Kushi Institute affiliates in London, Amsterdam, Antwerp, Florence, as well as in Portugal and Switzerland. Information on Leadership Studies is available from the Kushi Institute in Boston, Massachusetts.

OTHER PROGRAMS

The Kushi Institute offers a variety of public programs including an annual Summer Conference in western Massachusetts, special weight-loss and natural beauty seminars, and intensive cooking and spiritual development training at the Berkshires Center. Moreover, a variety of introductory and public programs are offered through an international network of over 300 educational centers in the United States, Canada, and throughout the world. The Kushi Foundation publishes a *Worldwide Macrobiotic Directory* every year listing these centers and individuals. Please consult the *Directory* for the nearest macrobiotic center or qualified instructor.

PUBLICATIONS

Michio and Aveline Kushi have authored numerous books on macrobiotic cooking, philosophy, diet, and way of life. These titles are listed in the Recommended Reading list and are available at macrobiotic centers, natural food stores, and bookstores. Ongoing developments are reported in the *East West Journal*, a monthly magazine begun in 1971 with an international readership of 200,000. The *Journal* features regular articles on the macrobiotic approach to health and nutrition, as well as related subjects. It is available at most natural food stores and by subscription.

Recommended Reading

Aihara, Cornellia. *The Dō of Cooking*. Chico, Calif.: George Ohsawa Macrobiotic Foundation, 1972.

_____. *Macrobiotic Childcare*. Oroville, Calif.: George Ohsawa Macrobiotic Foundation, 1971.

Aihara, Herman. *Basic Macrobiotics*. Tokyo & New York: Japan Publications, Inc., 1985.

Benedict, Dirk. *Confessions of a Kamikaze Cowboy*. Van Nuys, Calif.: Newcastle, 1987.

Brown, Virginia, with Susan Stayman. *Macrobiotic Miracle: How a Vermont Family Overcame Cancer*. Tokyo & New York: Japan Publications, Inc., 1985.

Dietary Goals for the United States. Washington, D. C.: Select Committee on Nutrition and Human Needs, U.S. Senate, 1977.

Diet, Nutrition and Cancer. Washington, D. C.: National Academy of Sciences, 1982.

Dufty, William. *Sugar Blues*. New York: Warner Books, 1975.

Esko, Edward and Wendy Esko. *Macrobiotic Cooking for Everyone*. Tokyo & New York: Japan Publications, Inc., 1980.

Esko, Wendy. *Aveline Kushi's Introducing Macrobiotic Cooking*. Tokyo and New York: Japan Publications, Inc., 1987.

Fukuoka, Masanobu. *The Natural Way of Farming*. Tokyo & New York: Japan Publications, Inc., 1985.

_____. *The One-Straw Revolution*. Emmaus, Pa.: Rodale Press, 1978.

Healthy People: The Surgeon General's Report on Health Promotion and Disease Prevention. Washington, D. C.: Government Printing Office, 1979.

Hiedenry, Carolyn. *Making the Transition to a Macrobiotic Diet*. Garden City Park, N.Y.: Avery Publishing Group, 1987.

Hippocrates. *Hippocratic Writings*. Edited by G. E. R. Lloyd. Translated by J. Chadwick and W. N. Mann. New York: Penguin Books, 1978.

I Ching or *Book of Changes*. Translated by Richard Wilhelm and Cary F. Baynes. Princeton: Bollingen Foundation, 1950.

Ineson, John. *The Way of Life: Macrobiotics and the Spirit of Christianity*. Tokyo & New York: Japan Publications, Inc., 1986.

Jacobs, Leonard and Barbara Leonard. *Cooking with Seitan*. Tokyo & New York: Japan Publications, Inc., 1986.

Jacobson, Michael. *The Changing American Diet*. Washington, D. C.: Center for Science in the Public Interest, 1978.

Kaibara, Ekiken. *Yojokun: Japanese Secrets of Good Health*. Tokyo: Tokuma Shoten, 1974.

Kidder, Ralph D. and Edward F. Kelley. *Choice for Survival: The Baby Boomer's Dilemma*. Tokyo & New York: Japan Publications, Inc., 1987.

Kohler, Jean and Mary Alice. *Healing Miracles from Macrobiotics*. West Nyack, N. Y.: Parker, 1979.

Kotsch, Ronald. *Macrobiotics: Yesterday and Today*. Tokyo & New York: Japan Publications, Inc., 1985.

Kushi, Aveline. *How to Cook with Miso*. Tokyo & New York: Japan Publications, Inc., 1978.

_____. *Lessons of Night and Day*. Garden City Park, N.Y.: Avery Publishing Group, 1985.

_____. *Macrobiotic Food and Cooking Series: Diabetes and Hypoglycemia; Allergies*. Tokyo & New York: Japan Publications, Inc., 1985.

_____. *Macrobiotic Food and Cooking Series: Obesity, Weight Loss, and Eating Disorders; Infertility and Reproductive Disorders*. Tokyo & New York: Japan Publications, Inc., 1987.

Kushi, Aveline, with Alex Jack. *Aveline Kushi's Complete Guide to Macrobiotic Cooking*. New York: Warner Books, 1985.

Kushi, Aveline and Michio Kushi. *Macrobiotic Pregnancy and Care of the Newborn*. Edited by Edward and Wendy Esko. Tokyo & New York: Japan Publications, Inc., 1984.

_____. *Macrobiotic Child Care and Family Health*. Tokyo & New York: Japan Publications, Inc., 1986.

Kushi, Aveline, and Wendy Esko. *Macrobiotic Family Favorites*. Tokyo & New York: Japan Publications, Inc., 1987.

Kushi, Aveline, and Wendy Esko. *The Changing Seasons Macrobiotic Cookbook*. Garden City Park, N.Y.: Avery Publishing Group, 1983.

Kushi, Michio. *The Book of Dō-In: Exercise for Physical and Spiritual Development*. Tokyo & New York: Japan Publications, Inc. 1979.

_____. *The Book of Macrobiotics: The Universal Way of Health, Happiness and Peace*. Tokyo & New York: Japan Publications, Inc., 1986 (Rev. ed.).

_____. *Cancer and Heart Disease: The Macrobiotic Approach to Degenerative Disorders*. Tokyo & New York: Japan Publications, Inc., 1986 (Rev. ed.).

_____. *Crime and Diet: The Macrobiotic Approach*. Tokyo & New York: Japan Publications, Inc., 1987.

_____. *The Era of Humanity*. Brookline, Mass.: East West Journal, 1980.

_____. *How to See Your Health: The Book of Oriental Diagnosis*. Tokyo & New York: Japan Publications, Inc., 1980.

_____. *Macrobiotic Health Education Series: Diabetes and Hypoglycemia; Allergies*. Tokyo & New York: Japan Publications, Inc., 1985.

_____. *Macrobiotic Health Education Series: Obesity, Weight Loss, and Eating Disorders; Infertility and Reproductive Disorders*. Tokyo & New York: Japan Publications, Inc., 1987.

_____. *Natural Healing through Macrobiotics*. Tokyo & New York: Japan Publications, Inc., 1978.

_____. *On the Greater View: Collected Thoughts on Macrobiotics and Humanity*. Garden City Park, N.Y.: Avery Publishing Group, 1985.

_____. *Your Face Never Lies*. Garden City Park, N.Y.: Avery Publishing Group, 1983.

Kushi, Michio, and Alex Jack. *The Cancer Prevention Diet*. New York: St. Martin's Press, 1983.

_____. *Diet for a Strong Heart*. New York: St. Martin's Press, 1984.

Kushi, Michio, with Alex Jack. *One Peaceful World*. New York: St. Martin's Press, 1987.

Kushi, Michio and Aveline Kushi, with Alex Jack. *The Macrobiotic Diet*. Tokyo & New York: Japan Publications, Inc., 1985.

Kushi, Michio, and the East West Foundation. *The Macrobiotic Approach to Cancer*. Garden City Park, N.Y.: Avery Publishing Group, 1982.

Kushi, Michio, with Stephen Blauer. *The Macrobiotic Way*. Garden City Park, N.Y.: Avery Publishing Group, 1985.

Mendelsohn, Robert S., M. D. *Confessions of a Medical Heretic*. Chicago: Contemporary Books, 1979.

_____. *Male Practice*. Chicago: Contemporary Books, 1980.

Nussbaum, Elaine. *Recovery: From Cancer to Health through Macrobiotics*. Tokyo & New York: Japan Publications, Inc., 1986.

Nutrition and Mental Health. Washington, D. C.: Select Committee on Nutrition and Human Needs, U.S. Senate, 1977, 1980.

Ohsawa, George. *Cancer and the Philosophy of the Far East*. Oroville, Calif.: George Ohsawa Macrobiotic Foundation, 1971 edition.

_____. *You Are All Sanpaku*. Edited by William Dufty. New York: University Books, 1965.

_____. *Zen Macrobiotics*. Los Angeles: Ohsawa Foundation, 1965.

Price, Western, A., D. D. S. *Nutrition and Physical Degeneration*. Santa Monica, Calif.: Price-Pottenger Nutritional Foundation, 1945.

Sattilaro, Anthony, M. D., with Tom Monte. *Recalled by Life: The Story of My Recovery from Cancer*. Boston: Houghton-Mifflin, 1982.

Schauss, Alexander. *Diet, Crime, and Delinquency*. Berkeley, Calif.: Parker House, 1980.

Scott, Neil E., with Jean Farmer. *Eating with Angels*. Tokyo & New York: Japan Publications, Inc., 1986.

Tara, William. *A Challenge to Medicine*. Tokyo & New York: Japan Publications, Inc., 1987.

———. *Macrobiotics and Human Behavior*. Tokyo & New York: Japan Publications, Inc., 1985.

Yamamoto, Shizuko. *Barefoot Shiatsu*. Tokyo & New York: Japan Publications, Inc., 1979.

The Yellow Emperor's Classic of Internal Medicine. Translated by Ilza Veith, Berkeley: University of California Press, 1949.

About the Authors

AVELINE KUSHI was born in 1923 in a small mountain village in the Izumo area of Japan. At college, she was a star gymnast. But her athletic career was cut short by World War II. During the war, she taught elementary school in her mountain district. After the war, she became involved in world peace activities at the Student World Government Association near Tokyo directed by George Ohsawa. In 1951, she came to the United States and married Michio Kushi. Along with her husband, Aveline Kushi has devoted her life to increasing awareness about macrobiotic philosophy. As co-founder of Erewhon, the *East West Journal*, the East West Foundation, the Kushi Institute, and the Kushi Foundation, she has taken an active role in macrobiotic education and development.

During the last twenty years in the Boston area, thousands of young people have visited and studied at her home in order to change their way of life in a more natural direction. She has given countless seminars on macrobiotic cooking, pregnancy and child care, and medicinal cooking for cancer, heart disease, and AIDS patients. She has been instrumental in arranging visits to the United States by teachers and practitioners of such traditional arts as the Tea Ceremony, Noh Drama, and Buddhist meditation.

Aveline has written and illustrated several books including *Aveline Kushi's Complete Guide to Macrobiotic Cooking* (Warner Books, 1985), *The Changing Seasons Macrobiotic Cookbook* (Avery Publishing Group, 1985), *Macrobiotic Diet* (Japan Publications, 1985), *Macrobiotic Pregnancy and Care of the Newborn* (Japan Publications, 1984), and *Macrobiotic Child Care and Family Health* (Japan Publications, 1986). The mother of five children and the grandmother of five, she resides in Brookline, Massachusetts and Becket, Massachusetts; and, with her husband, spends roughly half of each year teaching abroad. Her autobiography, *Aveline: The Life and*

Dream of the Woman Behind Macrobiotics Today, was published in 1988 by Japan Publications.

WENDY ESKO was born in upstate New York in 1949. She began macrobiotic studies in Boston in 1973, and, with her husband, Edward, pioneered macrobiotic education programs in the 1970s, including summer study programs at Amherst College in Massachusetts and annual conferences on the macrobiotic approach to cancer. She has taught macrobiotic cooking for more than twelve years, and is the former director of the Kushi Institute School of Cooking in Brookline, Massachusetts. She has co-authored several popular books on the subject of macrobiotics, including *Macrobiotic Cooking for Everyone* (Japan Publications, 1980), and with Aveline Kushi, *The Changing Seasons Macrobiotic Cookbook* and *Aveline Kushi's Introducing Macrobiotic Cooking* (Japan Publications, 1987). Wendy lives with her husband and seven children in Becket and teaches at the Kushi Foundation Berkshires Center in Western Massachusetts.

Index